P9-BIV-077

the healing code

the healing code

dermot o'connor

one man's amazing journey back to health
and his proven five-step plan to recovery

**HODDER
MOBIUS**

HODDER
HEADLINE
IRELAND

The information contained in this book has been obtained from reliable sources. However, it is intended as a guideline only and should never be used as a replacement for consultation with your regular physician. While every effort has been made to ensure its accuracy, no responsibility for loss, damage or injury occasioned to any person acting or refraining from action as a result of information contained herein can be accepted by the publishers or author.

Copyright © 2006 by Dermot O'Connor

First published in Ireland in 2006 by Hodder Headline Ireland
A division of Hodder Headline

First published in Great Britain in 2006 by Hodder and Stoughton
A division of Hodder Headline

The right of Dermot O'Connor to be identified as the
Author of the Work has been asserted by him in accordance
with the Copyright, Designs and Patents Act 1988.

A Hodder Headline Ireland/Mobius Book/paperback

3

All rights reserved. No part of this publication may be reproduced, stored in a retrieval system, or transmitted, in any form or by any means without the prior written permission of the publisher, nor be otherwise circulated in any form of binding or cover other than that in which it is published and without a similar condition being imposed on the subsequent purchaser.

A CIP catalogue record for this title is available from the British Library

ISBN 0 340 89815 1
Ireland ISBN (Including Northern Ireland) 0 340 89940 9

Typeset in Legacy by Hewer Text UK Ltd, Edinburgh
Printed and bound by Clays Ltd, St Ives plc

Every effort has been made to fulfil requirements with regard to reproducing copyright material. The author and the publisher will be glad to rectify any omissions at the earliest opportunity.

Hodder Headline's policy is to use papers that are natural, renewable and recyclable products and made from wood grown in sustainable forests. The logging and manufacturing processes are expected to conform to the environmental regulations of the country of origin.

Hodder and Stoughton & Hodder Headline Ireland
Divisions of Hodder Headline
338 Euston Road
London NW1 3BH

www.hhireland.ie
www.hoddermobius.com

Dedicated to my mother Mary, whose love has always been boundless, my father Joe, whose courage, strength and integrity are inspirational and to Grace, Alison and Faye who heal everything with a smile.

Acknowledgements

This book would not have been possible without the assistance and encouragement of many individuals to whom I would like to extend my sincerest appreciation.

I would like to thank the three wise men, Dr Sean Collins, Dr Vincent Carroll and Dr Richard Bandler for the knowledge and wisdom they have shared.

A special thanks to Paul McKenna, for his generosity and incredible support.

Deepest gratitude to Ron Downes, whose constant friendship has helped me more in life than he will ever know.

A special thanks to Robert Kirby, Rowena Webb, Ciara Considine and Teresa Hale.

Finally my thanks go to all my clients who have embraced the principles of this book. It is because of their inspiring and miraculous stories of health recovery that the true power of the Healing Code was revealed.

Contents

Foreword

When faced with life-challenging illnesses, there are a number of responses open to us:

- For many people in such circumstances, the natural response is one of resignation, even despair. However understandable this response may be, the harsh reality is that this approach will not help our chances of recovery – and will most probably hinder us.
- A second response is to put our faith entirely in the medical establishment – essentially delegating responsibility for our health and well-being to others. Modern medicine continues to make great strides and it would be foolhardy to ignore its benefits, but if we focus solely on modern medicine, to the neglect of other proven approaches to healing, we run the risk of fighting illness with one hand tied behind our back.
- The third approach, and the approach advocated in Dermot O'Connor's remarkable new book, is to harness all of the powers at our disposal in a powerful personal quest for wellness.

Dermot's path to health recovery weaves together the proven, timeless healing wisdom of the East with the latest discoveries in health psychology and medical science to form a seamless holistic approach to reclaiming our health. The result is the Healing Code.

In the pages of this book, Dermot reveals many wonders, ranging from the miracles of optimum nutrition to the powerful healing arts of medical chi kung and cutting-edge mind-medicine technologies for self-healing. But the most wonderful thing about Dermot's approach is this: it works! Focusing on the things that work – this is the guiding principle that has led Dermot to unravel the secrets of the Healing Code. No prejudices, no preconceptions, no gimmicks – just a relentless commitment to finding the truth about health and healing.

The reason for Dermot's honest approach is disarmingly simple: confronted with a life-challenging illness, Dermot simply couldn't afford to get it wrong. He could depend only on facts – tried and tested approaches, based on evidence and results. Dermot's journey has been an inspiring one. And the best part of the journey is the triumphant return, laden with riches that he is eager to share.

Now established as one of Europe's leading practitioners of Eastern medicine, including acupuncture and medical chi kung, Dermot has honed his unique sensitivity to therapeutic techniques that actually have health-giving value. Having dealt with therapists and holistic practitioners around the country, I recognise in the Healing Code an approach that is comprehensive, progressive and distinctly personal. Dermot's emphasis on using the proven elements of Eastern and Western medicine side by side is refreshing and astute, and I hope it will inspire the average person to experience for themselves the profound health benefits to be found in holistic therapies.

The Healing Code system is an eminently sensible, logical and practical plan of action for people who want to reclaim their health in the face of serious and life-challenging illness. Dermot sets out, step by step, the right way to do the right things. If you want to get healthy against the odds – and if you want to *stay* healthy – the Healing Code will prepare you for success. *Knowing* that you're doing everything in your power to win – that in itself is a potent sign of imminent healing. And that knowledge is only the first of the secrets of the Healing Code . . .

I commend this book to you, and I trust that your journey, too, will lead to healing, health and happiness.

Teresa Hale,
founder of The Hale Clinic

Introduction

'If there's one thing I say to those who use me as their example, it's that if you ever get a second chance in life, you've got to go all the way.'

LANCE ARMSTRONG, diagnosed with testicular cancer in 1996 and winner of a record-breaking seven consecutive Tour de France titles

This book will reveal many secrets. I promise that these secrets will heal, transform and revitalise your life. The book brings together the five key elements consistently used by men and women throughout history to successfully recover from a spectrum of life-challenging illness from heart disease to MS, diabetes and cancer. These elements encompass the Healing Code, a complete system, which is supported by medical science and guaranteed to enhance the resurgence of well-being.

Let us have no illusions: being diagnosed with a life-threatening illness is a challenge that requires an Olympian reaction. Anyone who succeeds in the battle against such an illness is no less a hero than any gold medallist, and success requires dedication and commitment. Those who succeed in this challenge may not get a place on a podium, but their prize is far more valuable than any gold medal. The prize is life itself.

When confronted with a diagnosis of a life-challenging illness, people will respond in differing ways. Firstly, many people take a hands-off or 'do it to me' approach. They deal with the emotional trauma of the diagnosis as best they can, but ultimately they rely almost entirely on medical interventions that can be made by their doctor or surgeon. They become almost like spectators and simply hope that their medical team will do the best they can for them. This would be like an Olympic hopeful who relied entirely upon the brilliance of his coach but didn't bother to train, eat the right food or develop the mental resilience necessary to compete.

A second common response is to react in a state of panic. The patient 'tries everything' and visits anyone who has been suggested as having a 'cure' to their illness. They may often try many legitimate approaches but will drop them unless a 'cure' is immediate. Although they may say that they have 'tried everything', in reality they have tried nothing. It would be like preparing for the Olympics by doing physical exercise for one day and not continuing because you didn't break any records on that day, and then deciding to change your diet for a few days, to see if that worked.

Logically, neither of these approaches will yield many Olympic medals, and yet when faced with the challenge of a life-threatening illness, many people respond in one of these two ways. However, those who have faced and overcome such life challenges have usually reacted in a manner similar to that of a successful athlete. Like the athlete who chooses the best coach he can get, the successful health recovery will involve following the best medical advice, together with optimum and proven approaches to mind, emotion, nutrition and exercise so that your body's own self-healing abilities are maximised.

Every element of the Healing Code is guaranteed to enhance your chances of winning that gold medal – a lasting health recovery.

The Healing Code – The Secret of Spontaneous Healing

Now let us begin with a mystery. A successful executive has been troubled by strange bouts of dizziness, numbness and slurred speech. Then suddenly he loses sensation over his entire body. After extensive medical tests the neurologist gives the dreadful diagnosis – an aggressive form of multiple sclerosis (MS), the 'incurable' and degenerative nerve disease. The news comes as a hammer blow. Dreams for the future are swept away, and the doctors advise him to brace for 'managed decline' – the heartless clinical term for the inexorable slide into dependency, disease and death.

At first he accepts the grim prognosis – with fatalism, futility and despair. He educates himself as to what MS could bring. As he reads of each symptom, he notices that they seem to seep into his very being, dragging him hastily towards disability.

However, after six months of deepest despair, his attitude changes, and by harnessing the power of the subconscious mind, he begins to move towards hope. In his mind's eye he creates a positive and vibrant self-image, which he moves towards with increasing confidence. Eight years after diagnosis he is back in the best physical and mental health of his life, symptom-free and without any trace of the illness. This is my story, and it is simply one of countless amazing healing stories that frequently appear to confound modern science.

Take Lance Armstrong, who in 1996 appeared to be on the threshold of a charmed life. A new American champion cyclist who seemed physically invincible was destined to become known the world over. Suddenly, out of nowhere, his entire life came crashing down at once when he was diagnosed with aggressive testicular cancer, which was spreading like wildfire through his body. His cancer had established itself in his abdomen, his lungs and even his brain. There were 11 masses in his lungs alone, some the size of golf balls. His brain was invaded by two malignancies, and he was given a less than 50% chance of surviving just a few months.

The mind and the body are inextricably linked, and how you think can promote or hinder the healing process. This as much as anything explains the miraculous recovery of Lance Armstrong in the year that followed. It was a challenging year during which he underwent a barrage of treatment, but it was not a year of depression, resignation or failure. He harnessed a powerful mental approach, optimum nutrition, emotional strength and exercise, and incredibly, in 1997, Lance was declared cancer-free. He had fought through the darkness, and now the brightness of success had returned.

Just two short years later Lance's body was back to a strength greater than he had ever known. Lance Armstrong cycled up the Champs-Elysées, through the streets of Paris, to claim victory in the 1999 Tour de France. His victories, both in athletic competition and health, were dramatic . . . and now complete.

Lance Armstrong was not supposed to be the champion of that year's Tour de France. His doctors really expected him to have passed from this world. But Lance paid no attention to that kind of thinking and stood triumphant over both cancer and the Tour de France. Lance has now won the Tour de France a staggering seven times.

You have within your possession the same tools and abilities to restore your health that Lance Armstrong, myself and countless others have used. This book will guide you through the process with clarity, conviction and certainty. This is not simply a book of theory; it is only through practical application of the programme in its entirety that the full benefits can be realised. Treat each chapter as a piece of the jigsaw and, trust me, the power to heal yourself will be revealed.

How This Book Is Structured

To help you quickly learn the powerful principles of the Healing Code, I have organised this book into seven distinct chapters. In Chapter One we will look at my own personal healing journey, some of the mistakes I made along the way and how I finally found the path to recovery.

In Chapter Two we will look at the psychology of health recovery. For more than a decade modern scientists have recognised that behavioural and psychological events can influence the immune system, but now new research shows that the immune system sends signals to the brain that dramatically alter neural activity and thereby affect everything from behaviour to thought and emotion.

As the mind is the first key element in beginning the Healing Code, we will look at what a belief system is and how it can affect our health. Most importantly, we will see how altering your beliefs can trigger recovery. Our belief system provides the motive for everything we do in life. To establish an effective recovery, it is crucial to create a clear and effective belief structure that enables your vision of this recovery. We will look at how the subconscious mind works and how it can be harnessed to maximise healing potential. We detail how breakdown occurs between the conscious and subconscious minds and how this connection can be re-established by removing subconscious obstacles to health recovery. This chapter reveals powerful mind-medicine techniques that dramatically enhance the self-healing process. There is also an explanation of how guiding thoughts can heal your body. This is the first step on your Healing Code journey.

In Chapter Three we reveal how emotional trauma and suppression affect our body, and consequently how emotional release acts to unlock our healing potential. At this stage of the programme we will deliver powerful techniques that will reclaim your emotional health and thereby turbocharge the self-healing process.

The latest scientific research reveals the intimate links between mind and body. The 'information substances', or the molecules of emotion, link a network that includes the immune system, which is designed to learn, to remember and to adapt. This means that we can, on a conscious and a subconscious level, communicate with our immune system, as our immune system communicates with the rest of us. All of our cells are linked in an intricate network of communication and emotion. Emotions influence immunity, and the immune system influences emotions.

The links between cancer and the suppression of emotion, particularly anger, between susceptibility to heart attack and an overly hostile personality, and between 'feeling happy' and having a high resistance to some viral infections are only some of the areas that have recently been illuminated by research. We will harness this knowledge to optimise your emotional strength for total health recovery.

In Chapter Four we demystify the alchemy of food with the Healing Code Nutrition Plan. The latest scientific research reveals that as much as 70% of all cancers are preventable by nutrition alone! Nutrition plays a critical part in the development and consequently the treatment of practically all illnesses. Whilst many conflicting 'diet' books exist on the market, there is an emerging consensus as to what nutrition elements are key to maintaining health and promoting health recovery.

Your body is a temple. Just as a once glorious temple will quickly lose its grandeur unless it is properly maintained, you need the right food and nutrients to restore your body. Your body is designed to renew and repair itself; the problem is that we often give it poor materials to do the task. This chapter reveals the foods necessary to revitalise your body, together with a sensible approach to implementing the Nutrition Plan.

In Chapter Five you will take control of the habits and behaviours that compromise the self-healing process. When faced with a life-challenging condition, it is no time for half measures. We will deliver an effective strategy that will help you conquer unhelpful dietary and environmental pollutants, including smoking and other factors that have a direct impact on your ability to recover health.

When we remove elements that compromise the body's self-healing process, your body is ready to win the battle for revival.

In Chapter Six you will learn the ultimate exercise healing system – medical chi kung. Chi kung, which means 'energy cultivation', is traditional Chinese medicine's most ancient system of healing and is considered by many to be its most powerful. It has been scientifically established that chi kung offers compelling benefits to those recovering from life-threatening illnesses from heart disease to cancer. These include improving heart and lung function, increasing blood supply to muscles and the ability to use oxygen, lowering heart rate and blood pressure, as well as increasing HDL cholesterol (the 'good' cholesterol). Conscious breathing, the technique employed by chi kung, is extremely powerful and there is a wealth of data showing that changes in the rate and depth of breathing affect the quantity and kind of peptides that are released from the brain stem.

This chapter will utilise powerful exercise, breathing and meditation techniques. It is supported by illustrations and will enable you to establish a personalised system of exercise that will most effectively combat your medical condition. This is the fifth step on your road to recovery.

Chapter Seven sets the scene for your Healing Code journey. Each chapter in this book delivers the optimum strategies for you to recover complete health. The renewal of health and well-being may seem at first like an intricate journey, but with the correct map we can find our way with sure and certain footing. As everyone is unique, so each journey will be different. Set out on this journey and ensure that you are relentless, have ambitious goals and have made no allowance for failure.

How Soon Will It Start to Work?

In my clinic, I have encountered many people who have been affected by ill health in what seemed like a heartbeat. However, for most of these people, there was a 'straw that broke the camel's back' moment, when it all 'fell apart'. When you analyse what had been happening in the lives of many of these people, you will often see long-term patterns of poor nutrition, emotional instability, poor physical exercise and high stress. When serious ill health struck, for many of these people it seemed like it was instantaneous: 'It came from nowhere.' The reality, however, is that it was probably a long time coming.

The good news is that the Healing Code will start to yield some benefits straight away. Diligent, continuous pursuit of the programme may lead to rapid results, or may take some time, but in the end, when health recovery is complete, it is likely to seem as instantaneous as the initial onset of ill health. But, you may ask, 'How can my body physically repair itself so quickly?' Well, let's take a look at the actual physical make-up of your body and see it for what it really is.

One of the miracles of the human body is that it renews itself, cell by cell, throughout your lifetime. Even when faced with life-challenging illness, our bodies are busy replacing damaged cells with new ones and are continuing their mighty effort to repair broken bones, cuts and bruises. The Healing Code will ensure that your body maximises its self-healing potential from the moment you begin implementing the programme.

How to Read This Book

'If I hear I forget; if I see I remember; if I do I make it my own.'
– Chinese proverb

This book is structured to guide you in a logical and clear manner on your path to health recovery. Throughout sections of the book you will be called upon to take action, make decisions and perform tasks. I encourage you to respond immediately on these occasions. This book works when *you* put the programme into action.

Take whatever time necessary to put the programme principles into practice. You may discover that some principles of the Healing Code are already familiar to you. That's fantastic! But ask yourself, 'Am I currently practising them?' If not, make a firm commitment to put them into action – now!

I recognise that any life change requires some mental resilience, even when you are in the best of health. It is for this reason that the first element of the programme is directed to ensure that your mind is ready to be well. Throughout the book you will also be given strong support in this mental aspect of the programme.

If you find yourself resisting taking some of the suggested action steps, or if practising some of the exercises doesn't seem to make sense to you, bear in mind that most resistance occurs when the need for change is greatest. Step up to this challenge and embrace the change with determination and the confidence that you are moving forward towards total health recovery.

So, let's begin our journey.

CHAPTER ONE

My Healing Journey

As usual I was running late. Always a night owl, I still felt groggy from lack of sleep. I jumped out of bed and rushed to get ready. No time for breakfast, I jumped into the car and started the morning off fighting through the city traffic. At 9.10 a.m. I was going to be late, but not so much that it would cause a problem. I hurriedly settled into my desk and made my first call of the day.

'Hello, itsch Dermosh O'Connor. Can I schpeak with Carlosh?' I slurred.

Colleagues turned round and laughed. 'What have you been drinking?'

I was just as surprised as they were, as although I had been up late, I hadn't been drinking at all. I considered that it was probably because I was tired and as soon as my head cleared I would be fine. I spent the rest of the day trying not to speak too much, as I did sound intoxicated. When I got home I went straight to bed and slept straight through from 7 p.m. until 10 a.m. the next day.

I woke up feeling much better. What a relief. I didn't know what had been the matter. I switched on the morning news to hear that 'New Zealand had lost rugby's Tri-Nations Championship for the first time since its inception.' That's a phrase I thought would put my speech to the test. I certainly couldn't have said that the previous day. Now, after much sleep, I felt confident. I paused and recited, 'New Zhealand losht rugbysh Tri-Nashions Championshipsh for the first time sinsch itsh incepshion.' My speech was certainly just as bad as the day before, or even worse. It was really quite strange and very frightening. Although I could think of the words, I couldn't shape my mouth correctly to pronounce them, no matter how hard I tried. Even after so much rest, I still felt really very tired and wondered what was going on. I was due to fly out on business to Germany the next day, and despite my difficulties, I decided to go ahead with the trip. What a complete disaster. Tough enough for a German audience to understand my Irish brogue, but when I seemed to have been drinking all night – no chance. At one point during my presentation I was literally struck dumb and just couldn't get any words out at all.

Two days later and I was still talking like I had had one too many to drink. I decided to do something that I hadn't done for years and go to see the doctor. She did a series of tests and decided that I ought to go straight to hospital. After I had presented the doctor's note at reception, I sat in the waiting room and prepared myself for a long wait in A&E. I was shocked by their level of urgency. The doctor came out straight away and said that I would be seen at once. I was sat on a trolley bed and told that they needed to do a CAT scan immediately.

'Why?' I asked.

'We think that you might have had a stroke,' she informed me.

'But I'm only twenty-nine.' I had such a shock that I had to lie down.

She pointed out that one side of my face was dropped. I knew that my grandmother was a relatively young woman when she had a stroke and she passed away within twenty-four hours. Should I now call my friends and family to say goodbye? I had always considered myself healthy. Sure, I caught a lot of colds, but nothing serious like this had ever happened to me.

After the CAT scan the doctor came back. 'The good news is that you don't have a brain tumour.' The potential causes of my speech problem seemed to be getting worse. I was glad that I hadn't realised a brain tumour was even being considered. The problem now, however, was that they didn't know what it was.

So over the next two weeks I underwent a barrage of tests. I had an MRI scan, which indicated lesions on my brain. But what did that mean?

'We also need to give you a lumbar puncture, just to confirm,' the consultant informed me.

'Confirm what? What do you think it is?' I protested.

'We think that it might be multiple sclerosis.'

I felt the blood drain from my face. I was familiar with MS. I would often say that I would take any health condition ahead of MS. It seemed to me to be one of the cruellest of all illnesses. Once it got a grip of you I believed that there was no release. You spent the rest of your life fighting a losing battle. That razor-sharp comedian Richard Pryor had MS and at this stage he was confined to a wheelchair and could barely talk. To say I was frightened was an understatement. I had my lumbar puncture and was discharged the next day. It was going to be a few weeks before the full test results came back.

By the time I had left the hospital my speech was back to normal. A friend mocked that I was never very clear to begin with and that he hadn't noticed the difference, but I was very glad to be out of hospital and feeling better. I convinced myself that nothing was wrong and vowed to spend the next few months getting back into shape and fit again. I started running again, something which I hadn't done in years.

Two weeks after leaving hospital I was still feeling well, but then it all went pear-shaped again. I woke up one morning and I had lost sensation all over my entire body. From the top of my head to my toes, if someone touched me with a feather or a nail, I would not have been able to tell the difference. There was also this strange sensation round my waist that felt like a tight band. I knew something was seriously wrong. Again I was on a business trip, this time in LA. When I got back to Dublin, I asked for an early appointment with the neurologist.

He started by doing a series of neurological tests. I had to push and pull against his arms. I was so determined to pass this test that I pushed him back so vigorously that he almost fell over. To my mind, I had performed all the tests admirably. But then he slowly took off his glasses and spoke.

'Listen, you have got MS. The tests came back and it's absolutely definitive.'

I could feel the blood drain from my face once again. No matter how much you think you are mentally prepared for the worst news, you can't really prepare for it. This had been my second attack in two months, which the neurologist indicated meant that MS was very active in my body. With the average being one attack per year, it suggested that this was a very aggressive form of the disease and my decline was likely to be swift. What could I do? I was told to go away and cry and to come back the following week with any questions.

The following week I returned with a long list of questions. I sat in the waiting room as people were called one by one to see the neurologist. I could see the varying degrees of decline as people before me struggled on walking frames and in wheelchairs. I wondered how long it would be before I was wheeling myself in for my appointment.

When I saw the neurologist, I worked through my list of questions, and any fragment of hope I had began to steadily fade. What could I do to help? Whilst medication could slow down the decline by 30%, nothing could halt MS indefinitely, and often the medication had side effects and sometimes didn't even work at all. What about other therapies? There was no evidence that any other therapies worked. What should I do with my diet? As there was no hard evidence that diet was a factor in MS, I should just carry on eating a normal diet. What had caused the disease? Was it anything to do with my lifestyle? The cause of MS was unknown, which made it more difficult to come up with a cure. In a nutshell I could take medication that might slow down my decline, but apart from that there was simply nothing I could do.

It was a dark, rainy day, but it couldn't be dark enough to reflect the deep gloom inside my head. My life seemed completely over, and truthfully I thought there and then that maybe it would be better if it was. Was I going to be a burden on somebody else? At this stage I had bought a number of books about MS. They seemed to be guidebooks to decline. One book in particular aimed to help readers 'cope' with MS and took me through the sequence of likely misfortunes that could befall me. The headings in the book ran 'Helplessness', 'Stress and MS', 'Accepting Help', 'Disability', 'Incontinence', 'Bowel Control', 'Neurological Pain', 'Musculoskeletal

Pain', 'Treating Pain', 'Living With Pain', 'Fatigue', 'Impaired Mobility', 'Sexual Problems', 'Spasticity', 'When Walking Fails', 'Long-term Care', 'Day-to-day Strain' and finally 'Death'! As I read each chapter, MS seemed to tighten its icy grip on my life.

Each morning I would wake with a sense that something was wrong but not knowing what it was. Then moments later the realisation of what had happened would hit me like a barge pole. I developed a morning ritual where I would test each of my faculties to confirm which had declined and by how much. Sure enough, as each day would pass, my legs seemed to be getting weaker, my eyesight seemed worse, my bladder more frequent, and I was developing pain sensations all over my body. I remember one time when my foot fell asleep and how I was stricken with fear. Was I about to lose my ability to walk? As feeling and movement came back into my leg, I was momentarily relieved, but soon enough my thinking went back to the worst. Had my foot just fallen asleep, or was it something more sinister? I had a constant sense that something dreadful was about to happen.

The odd thing about all of this is that I believed that I was coping well. When you are in the middle of chaos, it is often hard to know how well you are reacting to the situation. The ability to carry on functioning at all seems like an achievement. The worst thing about it all was the fear of the unknown. It was as if a giant was holding me in the palm of his hand. At any point the giant could decide to close his hand and crush the very life out of me. There seemed to be absolutely nothing that I could do about it. Sometimes the giant would close his hand slightly and I'd feel a symptom developing. Each time this would happen I would quickly be convinced that now was the moment of my absolute disintegration.

At this point I decided to tell very few people about my diagnosis. The more people who knew about my condition, the more I believed it would become a constant topic of conversation. I couldn't bear that. The constant conversation in my head was bad enough. For now, I wanted to control the impact of this diagnosis on my life as best I could.

But what had caused all of this? Of course I asked, 'Why me?'

Not in the sense that I was questioning divine will. I wondered what aspects of my life had brought this on. There were certainly things about me that were different from my friends and the people whom I knew. Could it be that one or perhaps all of the traits that were particular to me had contributed to the development of MS in my body?

I began a period of self-reflection, when I questioned many things about my thoughts, my life and myself. For instance, why did I have this burning ambition that could never be quenched? In my early twenties, when most of my friends were just having fun, I was working a full-time banking job and studying for two university degrees at the same time. Even though all my hours year round were filled with work, lectures and study, I was also looking for another academic course that I could begin working on simultaneously. Because my day was so full, I would often exercise by running or lifting weights well into the early hours of the morning, and afterwards I would literally collapse in my bed. Even when I didn't exercise, I rarely went to bed before 2 a.m. and often it would be closer to 4 a.m. It was as if life was a race for me and I had to achieve as much as possible as quickly as possible. I had no 'off' switch and never really recognised tiredness. Occasionally I never went to bed at all. This was a character trait I didn't see in anyone else I knew.

My job, too, made me somewhat different from most of my friends. For the previous seven years I had travelled all around the globe, working in over seventy countries. Frequently my work involved hopping in and out of different time zones, fighting off jet lag to perform under high-pressure conditions. Going to work with little or no sleep was again just a normal part of the job.

I also considered my earlier years. As a teenager I developed a very keen interest in sport. I liked to push myself to and beyond my physical limits. It was always important for me to train harder than team-mates, and I would often continue training after sessions had finished. I remember during one rugby training session we had to race by crawling commando style on elbows and knees across the gym. I won the race, but when I stood up there was a long trail of blood where I had ripped open the skin from my arms and legs. Although as an athlete I was really more suited to shorter distances, in 1988 I ran the Dublin marathon. When I had finished the race, I ludicrously decided to run a further three miles home. The very next day I was playing rugby. Of course there were athletes better than myself, but I rarely encountered anyone who would push themselves as hard physically.

Given that I was so interested in sports, you would think that nutrition was important to me. Sure, I ate a lot of good nutritious food; however, as well as all the good food, I also frequently gorged on junk food. The quantity of sugary food and drink I consumed was way above the norm. From an early age I had developed a sweet tooth, and this tendency had continued right into adulthood. By the time I was in my early twenties it was perfectly normal for me to drink as much as four litres of cola every day. It wasn't without reason that work colleagues called me the human dustbin. Even after eating a normal lunch, I would continue the afternoon by constantly munching on chocolate and sweets. Although if anyone had asked me about my diet, I still would have said that it was good. Simply because I did eat some good food, I didn't recognise that all this additional junk food was potentially being detrimental.

During this period of reflection I also looked at the way I handled my emotions. Like most people, I considered myself to be completely normal and emotionally healthy. However, I had to recognise that there was one trait that was particularly noticeable. Whenever I felt that I had suffered an injustice I would hold on to a huge amount of resentment and never let it go. For example, there was a time at school when my maths teacher had incorrectly marked my exam paper. I don't know what his motive was, but 15 years after it happened I still harboured huge resentment towards him. Whenever I would think about it, it was as if it had just happened to me. This was just one example, and although I was generally a cheerful person, I had stored a great deal of anger and resentment towards quite a few people.

Before my first MS attack in 1998 there were no obvious signs of any symptoms. It seemed to me that it had come completely out of the blue. Apart from a short time when I was a young child, I had never been to hospital, and it had been years since I had had any need to go to the doctor. So I had really considered myself to be quite healthy up until this point in my life. Again, this belief merited some reflection. Although I had hardly ever been to a doctor, I still had to recognise that I had a tendency to pick up a lot of colds and flu. On average I would catch around ten colds a year, and whereas other people would just shake their colds off fairly quickly, I would almost always develop a chest infection. I also had a constant sinus problem, and the notion of breathing in through my nose was something that I simply believed was not possible. I could never remember a time when I could breathe through my nose. As well as catching colds, I was also very susceptible to mouth ulcers. These I considered to be no more than a minor inconvenience, but now on reflection was this part of my body telling me that something wasn't working right? I'm sure my neurologist would not have recognised any link between the common cold, mouth ulcers and MS, but it seemed logical to me to look at my health holistically. Perhaps I had been getting clues along the way, which if I had recognised could have helped me to rectify my health.

At this point I was pretty convinced that I was doomed. All the 'experts' had left me with little or no hope, and mentally this had really taken its toll on me. By this time I was starting to think that taking my own life was a legitimate option, and I was not in the least bit scared of the rather harsh consequences. Suicide is a permanent solution for a temporary problem, but still I knew that I wasn't mentally in the right place to support my health in any respect. I knew that I had to make myself mentally stronger as quickly as possible. I hadn't contemplated that this mental strength would contribute to my health recovery. Mental toughness would just allow me to deal with my affliction in a more positive way as I began to fight an epic battle for survival.

During my career as a banking technology consultant I had been called upon to present to bankers in many countries throughout the globe. On many of those occasions my words were translated by an interpreter. I had understood that almost 90% of communication is non-verbal, and in furtherance of my professional career I began studying the use of language, physicality and communication on the mind. This had led me to the mind science of neuro-linguistic programming (NLP), created by Dr Richard Bandler, and I had built up quite a library of books and videos on the subject. If mental strength was going to be important for me at this point, I certainly had enough tools at my disposal to support this revival.

One of the videos in my collection was called *Supreme Self-confidence* by the world-leading hypnotherapist and presenter Paul McKenna. I began watching this on a daily basis. I should say 'attempting to watch', because within a few short moments of the opening sequences I would invariably drift away and only become conscious again at the end of the tape. Although I hadn't remained conscious, noticeable changes were certainly starting to occur. From the deepest despair, my attitude soon began to change. From somewhere within, a newfound hope emerged, which was the catalyst for a number of important and powerful changes I was about to make to my life.

One thing I did soon after this was get laser eye surgery. This short procedure corrected a vision problem I had had from early in my life. This did more than just correct my vision, however. It was positive reinforcement of the hypnotic suggestion of improved health. Through constant reinforcement of positive suggestions about my health something positive had happened within six months of my diagnosis. I went the entire day without thinking about MS at all. It simply didn't enter my thoughts!

Around that time I attended a lecture by Irish hypnotherapist Dr Sean Collins. Sean was conducting much valuable research on the effect of the mind on the body, and he had just completed his first book *Tipping the Scales*. In his work Dr Collins promoted the view that whilst making one change to your life might not be enough to conquer an illness, the cumulative effect of implementing a number of changes could be enough to tip the balance of the scales back in your favour. Sean's research trials were lending a lot of strength to this assertion, which to me made complete sense.

It is already scientifically acknowledged that almost 40% of all medical conditions are curable by the power of the mind alone. This includes everything from colds to cancer. Research trials eliminate this healing factor in order to establish if pharmaceuticals are clinically effective or not. Surprisingly, many drugs in regular use today have been passed as effective treatment that are just marginally more successful than the power of the mind alone. It struck me as strange that we are generally trying to eliminate from studies this mind-healing effect rather than trying to determine why the effect works for some and not for others. What if those who healed themselves with their mind could teach the rest of us what they did? What if the leading practitioners of hypnosis were there to guide us in this mind-healing process? I wanted to put together an arsenal of the best mind-healing techniques and so I sought out and trained with some of the world's leading practitioners of mind medicine. These included Paul McKenna, Dr Richard Bandler and the inventor of the strange but powerful system thought-field therapy (TFT), Dr Roger Callahan. I also worked with some of the leading practitioners of oriental shen-gong, or mind-work medicine, in China. Now I didn't just have access to some good mind-medicine teachers, I was working with the absolute best in the business and not only programming myself for health recovery but also gaining a host of positive life benefits.

As my mental state was now much stronger, I began to look at what other changes I could implement. Browsing the Internet, I looked for anything that might credibly contribute to my health revival. It soon became obvious that MS is a condition that many unscrupulous people are more than happy to take advantage of. There are thousands of Internet pages devoted to products proclaiming to be the miracle cure for MS. These 'snake-oil merchants' exist for almost every condition, and they are ready to take advantage of people at a time when they are feeling most vulnerable. Whilst browsing the Internet, I kept my head firmly on my shoulders and only took interest in suggestions that seemed logical, credible and had some solid supporting evidence. I soon discovered the work of Dr Roy Swank. Dr Swank believed that food and particularly fat intake were important factors for MS and he had designed an eating plan specifically for people with the condition. Dr Swank, a neurologist from Oregon, had conducted 50 years of research and worked with almost 5,000 people with MS. He had found that people who stuck rigidly to his low-saturated-fat, non-processed-food regime fared much better than those who continued with their 'normal' food intake. In fact, those who commenced the diet soon after diagnosis were still perfectly healthy after 35 years. I resolved to change my eating habits immediately, lock, stock and barrel.

Something that helped to motivate me considerably at this time was when I told a close friend of mine about my diagnosis. He had rather bleakly asked me how worried I was about possible future disability. Then when he walked to the bathroom I noticed how this man, because of his weight problem, was 'disabled' already, but he didn't even recognise it. Eating properly was something that I should do whether I had MS or not. Whilst at that point 'science' may not have been able to prove that nutrition was a factor in MS, I still was convinced that eating the right food had to improve my overall health.

Within three weeks of changing my eating habits I began to notice some dramatic changes in my health. Within just a few days my nose had begun to run profusely, but this was different from any other time when I had sinus trouble. My sinuses were beginning to clear, and this continued for a full four weeks, after which I could breathe clearly through my nose for the first time in living memory. The energy I had was hugely increased, such that I only now realised that I had been living with less than optimum energy for many, many years. There were other, more subtle changes. My thoughts got clearer, my memory improved, and I started to sleep better. Also, the numbness sensations that had been left in my body from the previous MS attack started to wane and finally disappeared.

So the food that I was putting into my body was now purer than ever before, and my body felt the better for it with each passing day. Of course, almost thirty years of poor eating habits do not get erased overnight. It was clear that whilst these dietary changes were hugely positive in the short term, I would continue to reap the benefits the longer I continued to eat well. So if the food I had been putting into my body had been a factor, what about other toxic elements?

One thing that always troubled my logic was the use of mercury in dentistry. How could it be safe to use one of the most deadly substances known to man in everyday dental procedures? There is a growing body of scientific evidence that shows ominous links between dental mercury and many serious illnesses, including MS. I decided that this deadly poison had to be removed from my body. Every time I chewed, brushed or ground my teeth some of this mercury was being released as vapour, which I was inhaling. How could this be helpful? Because my diet had been so full of refined sugar, it wasn't surprising that I had a lot of amalgam fillings in my mouth. So, over the course of a number of weeks I had toxic amalgam removed from my mouth by a dentist who specialised in the procedure.

Although I live in a city where I was obviously exposed to high levels of pollution, as best I could I reduced my exposure to toxins such as those contained in detergents and deodorants. I noticed my energy levels beginning to increase to even greater levels.

I was about to put this increased energy to good use and decided to get back to the gym and start exercising again. I commenced a full programme of training designed to increase both my strength and aerobic fitness. On my first day back I was surprised by just how unfit I had allowed myself to get, but within a few short weeks the improvements were considerable. I was significantly and measurably stronger, and my stamina had steadily increased. Of course, this brought improvements to my health but also a further boost to my confidence. With MS there are a lot of unanswered questions, and sometimes it isn't clear whether you are improving or not. Because my strength and stamina were being monitored, I could say with complete certainty that my physical strength and fitness were improving. I promised myself that these improvements would continue for years to come.

Alongside the already considerable changes that I had made, I also reawoke my interest in acupuncture and Chinese medicine. Following a rugby injury when I was 19, my knee had suffered some severe ligament damage that had meant that I couldn't play for three years. This was despite extensive physiotherapy and prolonged periods where my knee was completely rested. Finally, my sports doctor and physiotherapist told me that my injury would require surgery and that would carry the risk that my knee could even be left worse off. As almost an act of despair, I decided to visit a local acupuncturist to see if he could help. After just two treatments my knee seemed almost perfect, and astonishingly I was back playing rugby again within a month of my first session. This to me was a miracle that I would never forget. Now, after my MS diagnosis, I felt more than willing to make myself available for yet another miracle.

I went to my acupuncture and Chinese medical practitioner who asked me a series of questions about my health and my lifestyle. Based upon these, he developed my profile and prescribed a series of acupuncture sessions combined with herbal medicine. Not satisfied with just receiving treatment, I soon began studying these ancient oriental healing arts. My research into the Chinese medical view of MS was deeply enthralling. Although oriental medicine to the layman may seem almost mystical, it is in fact a deeply pragmatic and complete system. Chinese medicine was developed by observing how human behaviour, food intake, emotions and environmental conditions affect the body. Through thousands of years of observation Chinese doctors have been able to build up a thorough understanding of how patterns of illness manifest. If a Chinese doctor observes one simple symptom, such as dandruff or brittle nails, he is able to predict a whole variety of other symptoms, not because of any mystical ability but because he knows how these symptoms tend to correlate with other symptoms through a good understanding of Chinese medical patterns.

When I looked at the patterns associated with MS from a Chinese medical perspective, it was almost like reading my own life story. It predicted my diet, my lifestyle and my eating habits. It even predicted the weather conditions that would tend to prevail where I lived. There had to be something more in this. Furthermore, everything that was suggested in Dr Swank's diet was supported by Chinese medical theory. In 2000 I wrote an article for the MS Society, which drew together some of the beliefs that Chinese medicine held about MS. These included environmental factors, eating habits, emotional issues and exercise. A number of scientific studies carried out since 2000 began to lend support to many of these Chinese medical theories, and I was soon invited to give talks for the MS Society.

So by combining acupuncture, mind medicine, nutrition, detoxification and exercise, how was I after six months? I had lost a lot of body fat and was back to my optimum weight, I was measurably fitter, faster and stronger. My sinuses had cleared, and my vision following surgery was perfect. My energy was higher than I had ever known it before, and I had increased mental clarity. In fact, not only was I symptom-free, but I was in the best physical shape that I had experienced for almost ten years before I was diagnosed with MS. I now wanted to perfect these keys to health recovery.

I began to wonder if going to the gym was the optimum form of exercise that I could take. As I progressed in my study of Chinese medicine, I soon learned of one branch of the system called medical chi kung. Chi kung is Chinese medicine's system of exercise and considered by many to be one of the oldest forms of oriental medicine and also, perhaps surprisingly, the most powerful. If acupuncture and herbal medicine had contributed to such a surge in my health, then chi kung was something that I simply had to experience. Although chi kung is perhaps one of the most widely practised forms of exercise (remember, almost one in four people is Chinese), it is often very difficult to find a good practitioner who has a thorough understanding of chi kung. Unfortunately, this includes people who have been teaching chi kung for years. I began my quest to learn chi kung from some of the world's leading masters, which brought me to teachers from all over China and to knowledgeable and gifted exponents in the US. I spent time working and learning in Xi Yuan Hospital in Beijing, which is considered the leading Chinese medical hospital in China.

Although I had also studied chi kung in Europe, when I encountered the true masters of this great art, the difference was colossal. When performed with the correct mental intention, simple exercises can alter the way you feel physically and mentally in a very short space of time. I witnessed very sick people at Xi Yuan Hospital literally move, breathe and meditate themselves back to health. More than that, I personally experienced a growth in my own stamina, and I was now physically stronger than at any other point in my life. These simple exercises, which could be learned in a matter of hours, had the capability to restore health to practically anyone who practised them. It is not surprising that leading medical universities are now researching this powerful healing system's effectiveness at treating a wide variety of conditions, with some staggering results.

So the foundations of the Healing Code had been revealed. But how effective is it when put into practice by other people? It wasn't long before it became very clear the Healing Code principles were astonishingly powerful at treating practically all health conditions. I started to work with other people, and my clients' healing results were so amazing that it soon became apparent that my true vocation was in the medical profession. I left my career as a banking technology consultant and became a full-time practitioner. Word travelled fast and people were soon coming to me from far and wide. More and more we witnessed powerful health transformations with the Healing Code approach.

There was Sharon, who had optic neuritis caused by multiple sclerosis and was brought to my clinic because she had lost most of the vision in both eyes. After just three weeks she drove to the clinic herself with near perfect vision, and now, five years later, she is still in the best of health.

Then there was Phil, who was diagnosed with Dupuytren's contracture, a condition which affects one in six Caucasian men and causes the hand to start to form a claw. As a professional musician, this condition threatened his livelihood. His surgeon told him that in his vast experience he had never seen the condition reversing and that surgery, with all its potential complications, was the only option. Even then surgery would only temporarily increase mobility without addressing the underlying disease. After just a matter of weeks Phil's hand had improved to such a degree that his surgeon now informed him that surgery was no longer necessary. As far as the surgeon was concerned, this was a first in medical history.

Ciaran had been diagnosed with diabetes and high cholesterol and was warned that he was rapidly heading towards severe heart problems. Again within a few months of implementing the Healing Code, his blood sugar levels had normalised and his cholesterol had returned to a safe level. More than this, he had dramatically increased his health and vitality.

Joe had been diagnosed with Parkinson's disease 15 years ago. When he implemented the principles of the Healing Code, he saw his symptoms dramatically decrease. His tremors were so reduced that he was able to significantly reduce his medication. As a regular golfer, his handicap no longer reflected his physical ability and he started winning practically every competition he entered.

All health conditions seemed to benefit when the Healing Code was implemented fully. Dolores had suffered with severe migraines for almost twenty years. In fact, even when she wasn't suffering from a migraine attack she still had a constant lingering headache. Within less than a week her headaches disappeared and migraine was soon to become a thing of the past.

Declan had such severe sinus trouble that practically every month he spent a number of days at home unable to work and function normally because of the severe pain and discomfort. He also had fatigue and chronic digestive problems; he suffered with heartburn on almost a daily basis. After just a few short weeks of implementing the Healing Code, all of Declan's health issues were completely resolved. For the first time in over twenty years he knew what it was like to breathe through his nose again.

Eight years after my diagnosis my health has continued to improve year on year, and I remain symptom-free. Now a full-time medical practitioner, I have helped thousands of people implement the Healing Code and have witnessed first-hand how powerful the benefits are and how quickly they are seen. The first vital step is to understand and perfect the psychology of health recovery. So we begin implementing the Healing Code with a question: is your mind ready to be well?

CHAPTER TWO

Step One: The Psychology of Health Recovery – Is Your Mind Ready to Be Well?

The blood drained from my face when I was given the terrible news – acute, active, aggressive MS. Difficult to say how soon I would go downhill, but I had had two distinct attacks within two months when the average is only once a year, which suggested that I would go downhill rapidly.

'Go away and cry,' he said. 'Come to terms with the fact that you have this condition and that you are going to be disabled.'

I returned the following week and was told that there was no cure or any real way to halt the progression of MS. Only one drug existed and that only seemed to slow progression, and even then it didn't work for everyone. All in all, there was very little that could be done, and I simply had to accept and come to terms with my fate.

'What about diet?'

'No evidence that it helps,' he said.

'Is stress a factor? What about toxins?'

I was told that there was no hard evidence that these were factors and that I would probably be wasting my time and money if I tried to do anything about these issues.

It was a quiet journey home. I asked myself all the clichéd questions. Why me? I decided there and then that I would educate myself about this disease and cope as best I could. I bought every book I could find about MS and researched every possible symptom that could come to my door. Where optic neuritis occurs, sight is damaged, often leading to double vision, blurring and blindness. As each day passed, though I could still see, I could also detect the quality of my vision diminishing. Then I would check the strength of my legs. Again, I could still walk, but I was certain that the strength in my legs was decreasing. I noticed that in each area I focused my attention I seemed to be getting worse. I had soon developed a routine where I would check myself each day against any potential MS problem, and to my horror, I seemed to be getting worse in every respect. But then it occurred to me: was I actually causing my decline by my mental approach, and if so, could I equally use my mind to heal? I would have to change my attitude.

It was René Descartes who did most to establish the separation of mind and body in the world of medicine. Since Descartes's time medicine has generally held the belief that the mind (or soul) is distinct from the physical body. According to Descartes, the mind and soul were synonymous and were implanted into the human body by God. Conscious thought was the very essence of human existence and made man distinct from all other species. *Cogito, ergo sum* – I think, therefore I am.

Descartes believed that the mind was distinct from the brain, which was distinct from the body. This philosophy supported the existence of the soul and was therefore consistent with religious doctrine. Descartes's position was attempting to be both palatable to the Church and flexible enough to support the advancement of medical science. Until that time religion had held the belief that the body was the temple of the soul: any human dissections, and sometimes even operations, were fundamentally at odds with religious doctrine. A separate mind and body, he hoped, would facilitate medical development. Descartes was sailing close to the wind and was painfully aware of other scientists, such as Galileo and Giordano Bruno, who met their deaths for espousing beliefs that the Church held to be contrary to religious doctrine. Even though Descartes remained a Catholic all his life and firmly believed in the immortal soul, his works were still declared damnable by the Church in 1663.

It seems strange that Descartes's thoughts on the separation of mind and body have dominated medical beliefs until recent times, long after such threats of religious interference in medical advancement have subsided.

The World Health Organization defines 'health' as a 'state of complete physical, mental or social well-being and not merely the absence of disease'. Health is not something that you acquire; it is the process of being healthy. Health starts in the place that most people don't even think to look for it: your mind.

The Conscious and Subconscious Minds

The brain is absolutely central to the functioning of the body. Your brain performs two major types of function: those within your conscious awareness and those which we refer to as functions of the subconscious. Your subconscious mind is responsible 24 hours a day, 7 days a week for maintaining your heartbeat, breathing, digestion, repairing damage to your body, growing your hair and nails, controlling an enormous number of muscles to coordinate every single movement, as well as regulating your body's temperature, water content and sugar levels. In addition to all of these, it also has control of your body's regeneration, including growing a complete new skeleton each year, brand-new soft tissue every three months, a new liver every six weeks, eight square metres of new skin every four weeks and a new stomach lining every five days! In fact, 98% of the cells in your body are replaced every year.

So how can you use this information to make a huge improvement to your health? The first step is to sort out your central command centre, otherwise known as the brain. The key to doing this is to look at your belief system.

The Strength of Your Beliefs

People who recover from serious illnesses hold a strong core belief and a certainty that they will regain their health. For some, this manifests as a confidence in their medical team or medication, for others through a powerful belief in their own self-healing powers, and for others still simply through their religious faith. It is a fact that this attribute alone is enough to rapidly heal almost 40% of people dealing with illnesses – from the minor to the most serious.

Furthermore, when people take medication that does have a healing effect, almost 50% of that effect is attributable to the patient's belief in the medication.

This proven phenomenon has baffled scientists and is known as *the placebo effect*. When any drug company or research institute is trialling its medication, it must test this against the placebo effect. A placebo is an inactive substance or procedure used as a control in an experiment. The placebo effect is often misunderstood as a 'fake cure for a fake illness'. The opposite is in fact the case. Placebo drugs have been scientifically proven to be effective against a broad range of medical conditions, such as chronic pain, angina, high blood pressure, depression, schizophrenia and cancer. The placebo effect is a real and confirmed cure for a scientifically verified illness. This powerful healing effect is solely attributable to the power of the mind. The more the patient believes in the placebo drug, the more powerful and effective the healing response will be.

What is it that makes almost 40% of people respond to the placebo effect? What is it that 60% of people are doing wrong, and more importantly, what is it that 40% are doing right? The answer is down to your beliefs. Everything you do to improve your health, whether it's taking your medication, perfecting your nutrition or performing the exercises in this book, you must do all of these with a solid belief that they will produce significant health benefits. As Henry Ford said, 'Whether you think you can or think you can't, you're probably right.'

Your Health Vision

Muhammad Ali, known the world over as 'the Greatest', is generally accepted as the most supreme mental athlete in living memory. Ali won most of his fights long before he ever stepped foot in the ring. In preparation for a fight, how many times do you imagine Muhammad Ali contemplated ways in which he would lose a fight? The answer of course is that he would never contemplate losing a fight. He convinced his subconscious mind that he was invincible by repeatedly focusing his attention only on ways that he would win. He was so good at this that not only did he train his subconscious mind for victory, but he also trained his opponent's subconscious mind for defeat. He did this by writing and reciting poetry describing how and when in the fight he would beat his victim. Most of his opponents listened and played their role to enact these words in the ring. Remember, the nickname 'the Greatest' was, after all, given by the great man himself. Muhammad Ali even trained you and me! Muhammad Ali was brilliant at developing a clear, positive vision of success. This vision was so clear that making it happen became practically a formality.

Now ask yourself, 'What do I want in relation to my health?'

Many of us will answer this question by saying that we do not want a particular illness or health problem. You must remember that you always get more of what you focus on. So just as Muhammad Ali would only focus on winning a fight, we must redirect our focus and consequently our subconscious mind on our goal, which is full health, rather than 'no illness'. By being clear about the vision of health as opposed to the absence of illness, we are directed to move towards that vision. The more clearly and vividly we create that vision of health, the more accurately we train our subconscious mind to deliver it to our bodies.

So, let's create a solid vision of your healthy future by developing a 'well-formed outcome'.

Creating a Well-formed Outcome

Clear objectives cause us to focus our attention. Anyone confronting illness will often encounter confusion in their thinking. This can lead to a lack of clarity in what you want to achieve. Another common reaction among people with a serious illness is to become preoccupied with the disease. There is an old Chinese medicine saying, 'Wherever the mind goes, the body will follow.'

The following technique was developed by the genius mind of Dr Richard Bandler, the founder of neuro-linguistic programming (NLP), and will enable you to consciously train and direct your subconscious mind towards success.

The Well-formed Outcome Exercise

1. State your health goal in the positive. This means that rather than stating something like, 'I don't want to have a sore toe,' you would say, 'I want my toe to be strong and feel good.'

In a study, two rowing teams of similar ability repeatedly raced against each other. During the series of races they took turns at repeating two different mantras: 'We will win' and 'We will not lose.' Time and again the team that recited the phrase 'We will win' would come out as the victor.

The subconscious mind curiously deletes words like 'not' and will often direct you in the opposite direction to the one you really want to go. As an example, I want you *not* to think of an elephant! What picture did you create in your mind? You get the point.

Now choose your health outcome – and don't take any half measures. Make it a powerful and positive goal that fully captures the full health vision of your future. Write your vision below.

_____

_____

_____

_____

2. Next, I want you to be more specific about the outcome you want. In what way do you want to be healthy? What symptoms will have disappeared? State precisely how you want to be healthy again in a *positive* manner. Don't list your symptoms, but rather describe the manner of your health when these symptoms have gone – walking perfectly, breathing well, etc. Detail your outcome below.

_____

_____

_____

_____

3. Now I want you to answer the 'W' questions:
- What stage are you at in relation to this objective?

_____

- When do you want your objective to happen?

_____

- Where do you want this?

_____

- Who are the people who will benefit from this outcome?

_____

- What will achieving this outcome do for you?

_____

- What will you do with your life after you have achieved this outcome?

_____

4. Apart from medical tests, how will you verify that it has happened? Answer the following questions, which relate to your senses:
- What will you hear when you achieve it? What will you hear from your friends, family and medical team?

_____

_____

- What will you see when you achieve it? For example, smiles, tears of joy, your improved appearance in the mirror, a healthy complexion?

_____

_____

- What will you feel when you achieve it? For example, physical sensations of joy, love, happiness, excitement, pride, strength, relief?

_____

_____

– What will you smell or taste? Perhaps you will taste celebratory champagne?

_____

_____

5. Will you lose anything if you achieve this outcome? We will come back to this topic again later in the chapter. Think about what secondary gains your illness gives you that you will have to give up in order to achieve your chosen outcome. For example, bad habits, free time, attention, care from family and friends, control, comfort?

_____

_____

_____

_____

6. How will your life change after you achieve the well-formed outcome?

_____

_____

_____

_____

7. How will you start taking action to achieve your well-formed outcome now? For example, you will read and implement this book. What else will you do?

_____

_____

_____

Controlling the Voices in Your Head

From the moment we wake in the morning we begin a constant self-dialogue. For years I had a habit of being very harsh on myself. Whenever I would make a mistake I would talk to myself in the most ruthless manner. The problem that many of us have is that we aren't fully aware of the impact this dialogue has on our health and indeed our lives. In order to understand how we are thinking, we need to look at this self-talk. By becoming aware of the words and phrases you are using, the tone of voice and the intention behind those words, you will learn to understand the programming code of your brain. It is these words that are actually controlling your mind, and it is only by altering these words that you will reprogram your mind to self-heal.

Recognising Self-dialogue

1. Imagine that you have been given the task of looking after a new employee at a restaurant. This employee is nervous, and the boss has asked you to give this person as much personal encouragement as possible so that they settle in and become a successful employee.
2. Now imagine that this new employee has just dropped a glass on the floor and you have noticed that they appear very anxious. Close your eyes and imagine what words you would use to comfort this new recruit. Notice the tone of your voice and the positive intention of your words.
3. Now let's take a different perspective. I want you to imagine that *you* are the new employee at the restaurant. It is your first day and you are feeling very self-conscious and worried in case you make any mistakes.
4. Imagine that you have just dropped a glass and it smashes all over the floor. Notice what you would say to yourself. Notice the tone and the intention of your words. How is it different from the way you would talk to the other new recruit? Is it harsh, whereas the other was comforting?

The point is we do not allow anyone to talk to us in as harsh a manner as we talk to ourselves and yet it is this self-dialogue that rules our lives. Once you learn to change this dialogue, you literally change the course of your life.

Without being judgemental, notice your everyday inner self-dialogue. Do you recognise any of the following types of self-dialogue statements? 'There you go again; you do this all the time', 'Why do you always do that?', 'Why am I so stupid?', 'I feel so bad today', 'I'll never get over this', 'I feel like giving up', 'I'm such an idiot.'

It is estimated by leading psychologist Shad Helmstetter that 77% of all self-dialogue is negative and counterproductive. Whether you realise it or not, what you are putting into your brain in the form of this self-dialogue is what you will get back out. It affects our behaviour, feelings, self-esteem and ultimately our health. Your subconscious works hard to manifest whatever you tell it, and so by programming your mind with words and intentions, you are implementing the law of 'self-fulfilling prophecy'.

Constant thought and self-dialogue about ill health may be understandable in many circumstances, but it is practically always unhelpful. It is important to remember that the intention behind all of this self-dialogue is actually positive – to stop you making mistakes and to encourage you to do things better. But unless self-dialogue is conducted in a manner that is constructive and positive, then it will not benefit you at all. Now, I am not suggesting self-denial, because after all we are going to implement the Healing Code precisely because we have accepted that ill health has occurred. But if you allow yourself to focus your words and intention on the many different ways that your body can be unwell, guess what? You are training your subconscious mind how to manifest ill health. Bearing this in mind, it is worthwhile remembering that everyday conversations with your family and friends should not dwell on illness. We will look at this point in more detail later on in this chapter.

Your self-dialogue becomes a directive for your subconscious mind. Therefore, every time you make a statement that is negative about yourself or your health, you are directing your subconscious mind to make you become that person you've described.

Has the following ever happened to you? You lost your keys and went charging around your home searching in vain, repeating in your mind or out loud, 'I have lost my keys.' Then someone else came along and after saying, 'I'll find your keys,' they found them right where you had been looking? This is an example of how your subconscious mind has manifested an instruction you have unknowingly given it. You told your subconscious that you cannot find your keys and it obliged by making sure that you didn't – even when they were in front of you. This is known as a negative hallucination. It is a deep-trance phenomenon and shows how effectively your subconscious mind follows instructions.

The Language of Health

Now, bearing in mind how easily your subconscious is influenced, it is important to become selective about the words that you use to describe your illness. You said, 'I have lost my keys,' and that's what manifested. Similarly, if you say, 'I cannot get over this illness,' that too could act as an instruction to your subconscious.

I received a call one day from a man who described himself as being, like me, 'an MS sufferer'. I pointed out that I had no symptoms of MS and therefore I cannot be a sufferer, so I must be an 'MS enjoyer'. You must never describe yourself as an illness. Furthermore, if you describe yourself as a 'sufferer', what instruction do you think that is giving your subconscious mind? The same goes for words like 'chronic', 'acute', 'clinically confirmed', 'progressive' or 'terminal'. Any words that add strength or power to your illness must be removed from your vocabulary and replaced with words that more accurately reflect your recovery. We will look at this in more detail in just a moment, but firstly let's consider the following person's attitude to language and health.

Paul's Story

Paul came to my clinic after an MS attack had given him significant paralysis on the left-hand side of his body. He walked with great effort aided by a leg brace and walking sticks. He moved his left arm at a snail's pace.

As Paul was sitting down during the consultation, I foolishly asked him to remind me which was his 'bad side'. Paul confidently pointed out that he didn't have a 'bad side'. I asked him to explain. 'I have a good side and a recovering side,' he said. Wow, what music to my ears. After just one week Paul's arm was moving normally again, and after two further weeks he had thrown his walking sticks away, to the complete amazement of his neurology team.

This next exercise is a powerful way to reprogramme your thoughts and self-dialogue, which have a direct impact on your health. Many of us continuously indulge in unnecessarily negative self-dialogue. Why do we do this? Why continuously worry about things that might never happen? Why be fearful of worst-case scenarios that might never occur? Well, it's simply because we think we are helping ourselves to take action. But the reality is negative dialogue rarely pushes us into action, but rather creates an unresourceful state that often allows our worst fears to manifest. This exercise will turbocharge a powerfully resourceful state that will drive you towards better health.

The Three Steps to Reprogramme Your Mind for Healing

Step One – Thought Awareness

1. Sit comfortably on a chair. Closing your eyes, allow your body to relax and simply observe the flow of your thoughts for five minutes. Try to remember these thoughts. In the beginning you may notice that your thoughts relate to matters of everyday life; home- or work-related matters or worries may rush in on you. You must maintain the position of a silent observer, independently

watching the flow of these thoughts. Depending on your state of mind, this exercise will be difficult or easy. When difficulties occur, try to maintain your train of thought and observe attentively.

2. Start by practising this exercise twice a day, beginning for five minutes, and then each time you perform it extend the duration by one minute until you are observing your thoughts for ten minutes without digression. Once completed, you should be able to recall the train of your thoughts for the duration of the exercise.

3. As you practise, your thoughts will quickly become less chaotic. When you have mastered this exercise, your thoughts will have become slow, ordered and easily remembered. At that stage you can move on to Step Two.

Step Two – Thought Control: Empowering a Positive Self-dialogue

1. For the next stage of the exercise you will refuse to allow any negative self-dialogue to prevail in your thoughts. If any negative thought or statement such as 'I don't feel good' pops into your head, acknowledge the intent of the message, which in this case is that you want to feel good, and then immediately remove the negative statement from your mind.

2. Collect the negative thought and imagine literally cleaning it out of your mind. Visualise yourself wiping it off a white board and say, 'Erase,' in your head as you do so. Then replace the thought with a more positive equivalent such as 'I'm starting to feel good again.'

3. If you find yourself slipping up, avoid self-criticism, as this simply compounds the issue. Move on and practise this exercise until you can comfortably follow your thoughts for ten minutes without allowing any negative thoughts to invade.

Step Three – Thought Mastery: the Seven-day Healing Code Mental Reprogramme

You are now ready to move on to the final and most empowering stage of this exercise. You will learn how to retain a consistent state of mental positivity, which will have a direct impact on your physical health and well-being. By developing the habit of positivity you will become stronger – mentally and physically.

1. Over the next seven days refuse to dwell on any negative self-dialogue. This is to be practised throughout your day. You will reject all negative thoughts the instant they attack. Each such thought must be reframed, whereby it is transformed from a negative thought to become a positive thought, or else just rejected completely.

2. When you find yourself focusing on any negative self-dialogue, immediately use the 'Erase' method practised in Step Two. For these seven days you will train your mind to focus on positive solutions. As soon as you are confronted with a mental or physical challenge, immediately focus your intention on what you want the solution to be.

3. If you slip up and find yourself dwelling on negative self-dialogue for any length of time, accept that you need to continue to work on this exercise and begin the seven-day Healing Code Mental Reprogramme from scratch. Because consistency is a key component of the exercise, it is important to begin at day one again if you do slip up. This will ensure that at the end of the seven days, your mind is repatterned to consistently move towards positive self-dialogue and as a result physical healing.

Change Your Words and Change the Way You Feel

We touched on the importance of avoiding regarding yourself as a 'sufferer' and of using negative terms to describe your condition a little earlier on. Now we are going to look at this in more detail.

In a culture where success can be resented and failure celebrated, it often doesn't do to acknowledge happiness in any way. Our brothers and sisters on the other side of the pond do not seem to have the same stifling problem. How often when you are asked, 'How are you doing?' do you respond, 'Not too bad' or 'It could be worse'? What's wrong with using words like 'outstanding' and 'fantastic' to describe your day? When you are healthy and you use negative language, it trains your subconscious to not expect to have too great a day. As we know, what our subconscious expects is generally what we get. However, when you are not in full health, using language like this can have more serious consequences and can truly affect your powers of recovery. It is therefore important that from now on you get used to phrasing things in the most positive manner possible. And get this, I want you to phrase things even more positively when you don't feel totally fantastic – **just yet**.

Remember that we are not talking about denial. When you need medical attention to assist in your recovery, take it. We are simply talking about phrasing things in the most positive manner possible to train our subconscious to help manifest positive outcomes.

Take a moment right now to write down some of the words and phrases that you have frequently used in the past to make yourself feel horrible. At the time you may not have realised that this was going to be the effect, but now you know better. Words like 'depressed', 'angry', 'in pain', 'anxious'. When you have compiled a full list of the words that you have frequently used, come up with alternative words and phrases that change the emotional intensity. For example, 'depressed' changes to 'on the way back', 'angry' changes to 'irked', 'pain' changes to 'uncomfortable'. When you find yourself using a word or phrase that has strong negative intent, add it to your list and again find an alternative word or phrase.

To get you started, here are some ideas:

Negative word	Changes to
aching	niggling
acute	temporary
afraid	uncomfortable
alone	waiting for a friend
annoyed	irked
anxious	restless
chronic	frequent
disturbed	moved

exhausted	gathering energy
failed	moving towards success
frightened	challenged
helpless	welcoming support
hopeless	needing encouragement
hurting	uncomfortable
lonely	bored
nervous	expectant
not too bad	fantastic
out of control	making changes
overwhelmed	in demand
painful	uncomfortable
scared	eager
sick	recovering
stressed	energised
traumatised	moved to action
useless	not required

Writing Your Story of Health Recovery

We bring meaning to our lives through stories. Stories have a beginning, middle and an end. They have a structure and a logical flow, where things happen that cause other things to happen. We are used to thinking in stories and when we construct our image and understanding of the world we live in, we construct a story to make sense of it.

Scientists have become intrigued by the manner in which people with illnesses construct stories about their health. Leading physician Eric Cassell has contended that we commonly make a mistake in confusing the ideas of pain and suffering. Two people may have equal amounts of pain, but one may suffer a great deal whilst the other hardly suffers at all. The difference, Cassell concludes, lies within the stories that each patient constructs around the pain.

A story about suffering is one of isolation, pain and hopelessness. But the key point is that even when extensive and successful medical treatment is given, suffering may persist unless the story changes. Likewise, the suffering may disappear if the patient finds a way to change the story. It is therefore important that you can see and construct your health-recovery story.

Your Health-recovery Story

Construct a short story about you and your complete health recovery. Whilst basing the story on the existing facts of your case, make sure to present the story in a positive manner, progressing logically until the story concludes when you are back to enjoying full health and living a happy, fulfilling life. It is helpful to include some positive meaning behind your illness. When the meaning of the illness becomes more positive, then a spontaneous healing response is more likely to occur. How did your illness bring you to make changes in your life that made you happier and more fulfilled?

Let your imagination take you into a future where health, love and happiness are in complete abundance. Take the time out now to write your story. Do it now!

Altering the Hypnotic Effect of a Traumatic Diagnosis

Many people visit my clinic with what are considered serious illnesses. From my experience, before we can start treating these people we frequently have to address the trauma of the diagnosis and prognosis given to the patient by their doctor. It might surprise you that most therapeutic hypnotherapy is not about putting people into hypnotic trances. In fact, hypnotherapy is more about taking people out of a trance. During that moment when diagnosis is revealed, many people unknowingly enter into a trance-like state in which the patient's subconscious receives hypnotic suggestion regarding their health. The greatest hypnotherapist of the modern era, Milton Eriksson, defined hypnotic trance as 'the loss of the multiplicity of the foci of attention'; in other words, your attention goes from many things to one single thing. When your doctor is informing you about your prognosis, I guarantee you aren't focusing on what you are going to have for dinner. You are therefore by definition under a hypnotic trance. It's also why you feel dazed afterwards.

The trauma of this message can overactivate the sympathetic nervous system and leave the patient caught within a biological emergency pattern; they experience a constant sense of trauma and crisis, which in turn can have a deep impact on their health. Modern research has found that prolonged activation of this stress response, especially in the absence of physical outlets, such as vigorous physical exercise, may lead to a variety of ailments, from chronic indigestion, ulcers and high blood pressure to a build-up of cholesterol, aggravation of diabetes and lowered immune functioning. It is also known that extreme and violent shock from fright can lead to various phenomena, including sudden cardiac arrest, which pioneering neurologist and physiologist Dr Walter Cannon described as the likely cause of voodoo death. Voodoo death is the phenomenon in Haitian culture in which the 'witch doctor' is seen as such a figure of authority in his community that when he predicts someone's death by 'pointing the bone' at them, the person believes in his abilities and power with such conviction that he or she actually dies.

Let me say up front that doctors and medical consultants do fantastic work and should be applauded and appreciated for the great work that they do and the many lives they help. Of course they are obliged to inform you about your health. However, the fact of the matter is, if you have felt traumatised by the manner in which your diagnosis has been revealed to you, then that in itself may have a detrimental effect on your health and must be addressed. If this has happened to you, practise the following exercise ten times or until you no longer feel the same level of discomfort when you recall the moment of your diagnosis. Repeat the exercise if there were several instances of traumatic interaction with your doctor.

Breaking the Curse

Close your eyes. Picture in your mind the time you were told about your illness. Notice the image itself as a picture. If you close your eyes, you should be able to point to it. Notice the colours and size of the picture and hear the voice of the doctor. Notice the emotional effect that this is having on you.

Now drain the colour out of the picture so that it becomes black and white. Give the picture a silly soundtrack (my favourite is *Chitty Chitty Bang Bang*) and notice everyone in the picture moving in time to the music. Change the voice of the person telling you about the illness so that they sound like a squeaky Mickey Mouse or Sylvester the Cat. Now shrink the picture so that it is much, much smaller. Feel yourself starting to laugh at the silly voice and at what is being said. Now notice the change in the emotional effect that this new picture is having on you.

The reason this works is because your emotional response does not come from the person you are thinking about; it comes from the manner in which *you* are thinking about that person. You can change that. It is your mind, and you can have a choice about how you use it. This is an incredibly liberating realisation.

What to Look For In Your Medical Team

So, as you can see, the interactions you have with your physician can have a direct impact on your health. Remember, it is your health and you are the customer. If you are not getting the healthcare you deserve, this should be addressed. Exercise whatever healthcare options you have, and always look for the following qualities in your healthcare provider:

1. **They are prepared to take the time to explain how you will recover your health.** Having a good understanding of your health issue is an important element in enabling your subconscious to unleash its 'inner pharmacy'. The physician should therefore be willing to spend time explaining what the precise issues are and how your body will work to heal itself, with or

without clinical intervention. It is important that this explanation is delivered in a manner that is easily understood and jargon-free. You should not be intimidated in any way and should be comfortable asking any questions that you may have.

It is therefore also important that you make yourself available and invest your time in establishing this vital element of the healing relationship.

2. **They make you feel cared for as a person.** The perception that you are receiving care is another important element in helping you to unleash your own self-healing. This is based on feelings and instinct. Does the physician's bedside manner give you the impression it matters to him or her that you will be well again? Do they ask questions and want to know more about who you are? If so, the chances are that they truly do transmit a sense of care. The golden question is 'Do you *feel* better after speaking to them than you did before?' Because of the growing pressures placed on doctors in hospitals, where their workload is often overwhelming, it is understandable that this aspect of the interaction sometimes suffers. This is where there is a role for the complementary therapist, who can step in and support the caring role within healthcare.

3. **They give you an enhanced sense of mastery and control over your condition.** The gifted physician will give you a greater sense of being in charge of your life and your health. They should make you feel that you and he or she are in a true partnership working to restore your health. As a partner, you should get to make all the important decisions yourself. You will get good guidance, support and advice from your physician but will not feel dictated to. On occasions when you need additional decision-making support, your physician will take the reins, but you will take them back as soon as you are ready.

This is your life and the truly skilled physician will endeavour to give you as much power and control over your destiny as possible.

With care and encouragement, you will again take charge of your own life. As the ultimate goal is to make you healthy, the physician should also be empowered by your taking greater responsibility for your own health.

What You Talk About Is What You Think About

When I informed my friends and family about my health challenge, I also told them that I was still the same person and that I hadn't become the illness, so generally I wouldn't wish to talk about MS. Many of my friends told me afterwards that this was very helpful, as many of them felt an obligation to bring up the subject of my illness and it removed this task from their shoulders. There will be a few exceptions to this, and it is very important to share your feelings and vent your emotions, as we will discuss in Chapter Three, but it is also important not to dwell on illness. It must never be allowed to become the dominant and only topic of conversation, lest you unknowingly train your subconscious mind to support the very manifestation of that illness. The subconscious mind is very good at carrying out instructions. Fortunately, we can also use this to our advantage.

What many people do not realise is that they themselves are the architect of their thoughts. Of course, events happen in our lives from moment to moment that influence our thoughts, but importantly, it is not what happens to us that matters, but rather the perception of what happens to us. Take, for example, two people who survive a car accident. One is traumatised by the incident and has absolute conviction that he cannot function normally in his life again. The other firmly believes that he has been saved by divine intervention and vows that he will live his life to the fullest from that day forward. Both may turn out to be correct about their respective futures, which of course are remarkably different. But what has been the difference? Whilst the actual accident was the same for both parties, their perception was very different and has resulted in two differing outcomes – one very positive, and one very negative. The point is this: it's not the cards that you are dealt, it's how you play those cards. Although you may not be able to alter actual events that have happened, you can change your perception of those events. The exciting thing is that when you change your perception of past events, you by definition instantaneously change your future.

What You See in Your Mind Is What You Will Get

We think in words and pictures. We have already looked at the importance of maintaining a positive self-dialogue and positive vocabulary even in everyday communication. Equally important is to have a positive self-image that you move towards with ever increasing certainty. The following exercise trains your brain to envisage a complete health recovery. Just as an athlete visualises sporting success, and then frequently goes on to achieve it, you will create a vision of a full and lasting health recovery, which you will use as your goal.

Practise this exercise every day.

Reprogramming Your Self-image for Health

1. Sit comfortably on a chair. Allow your eyes to close as your body starts to relax. With each breath, feel your body relax more deeply.
2. Now, imagine seeing yourself completely healthy and invigorated and standing right in front of you. This is your true self.
3. Take some time to notice the characteristics of your true self. Notice the way you stand confidently, breathe, smile and move. Notice the way the true healthy you interacts with others.
4. Now, step inside your true self. See what you can see through bright, healthy eyes. Hear through the ears of your true self. Breathe comfortably and feel relaxed as your true self and notice just how good it feels to be strong and healthy.
5. Finish the session by allowing some time to visualise just how great your life will be as you live it as your true self.

Realigning Conscious and Subconscious Goals

Everyone who visits my clinic consciously wants to *be well*. It may at first seem strange that these same people could also subconsciously need the opposite. How can this polarisation of objectives occur within the same person? How can something painful fulfil a need? Let's look at a simple example. When a child falls over, he often looks to his mother before he 'decides' if he is hurt or not. Why is this? Perhaps the first time he fell over his mother rushed over and hugged and kissed him. If he cried, her hugs became stronger and a bigger fuss was made. He may even have got ice cream! Now, subconsciously, the child has learned to associate pleasure, in the form of his mother's hugs and ice cream, with the pain of falling over – so he tests it out by falling over again and again, and lo and behold, the same thing happens each time. So it's established: falling over equals lots of hugs. Any behaviour that fulfils a positive need, such as gaining love, granting attention, allowing us to have control or allowing us to have freedom, has the potential to become a need of the subconscious mind. Whether this behaviour is good or bad for our health is almost irrelevant. Once the need is met, the subconscious mind is satisfied.

It is worth remembering that our subconscious mind is more or less developed by the age of two years. Therefore in many ways we are driven and motivated by this two-year-old person living within ourselves. The important point to remember is that we are talking about the subconscious mind. The person consciously wants to be well, so it's not as simple as telling the person to 'get a grip' or to 'pull your socks up'. We have to communicate to the subconscious mind in more discreet ways. In order to do this, we need to ask some fundamental questions of ourselves.

This next exercise allows you to address the aspects that could be causing you to subconsciously gravitate away from health.

Subconscious Realignment Exercise

Step One

Begin by asking some questions of yourself and your illness. Try to be objective and treat yourself and the illness as if they relate to someone else. What benefits could this illness have given the subconscious mind that the conscious mind simply isn't aware of? Make a list and write them down. Does it mean getting care that has been longed for? Does it mean finally being listened to? Does it mean not having to work in a hated job? Whatever is relevant, take the time to write the list down *now*. Make the list comprehensive and complete.

Step Two

Now come up with alternative ways in which these benefits could be realised *without* having any detrimental effect to your health. For example, if you hate the work you do, a simple alternative to being sick would be to change job. Importantly, you don't have to do anything about achieving these new goals at this point; all you have to do is write the potential alternatives down.

So, for example, if in Step One you identified that this illness gained love and attention, in Step Two you could write that an alternative way to get this love would be to develop a more loving and fulfilling relationship and to connect with other people.

Take the time to go through all the potential secondary benefits that the illness grants you. With this exercise you are using your conscious mind to help your subconscious mind to see alternative ways to fulfil its needs without having to place any strain on your health.

The Power of Intention

The word 'intention' has many meanings. For our purposes, intention means stretching or bending the mind towards a goal or aspiration.

We have learned how to reprogramme our minds towards health by enforcing a consistently positive self-dialogue. However, it is worth remembering that the important thing is not only the words but also the power of belief and intention behind those words. Through practice we can learn to strengthen the power of our belief and intention so that as well as using positive words you also have strong, positive intention guiding you towards positive health resurgence.

A fundamental principle of intention is that ultimately our thoughts can create our reality. What we focus on in our minds is ultimately shaped in what becomes our reality. If we intend on speaking to a friend in our minds first and believe that we will soon meet this person, will it happen? Well, very often it does. As biologist and author Rupert Sheldrake points out, 'The idea of the extended mind makes better sense of our experience than the mind-in-the-brain theory. Above all, it liberates us. We are no longer imprisoned within the narrow compass of our skulls, our minds separated and isolated from each other. We are no longer alienated from our bodies, from our environment and from other people. We are interconnected.' The patterns of our thoughts can therefore shape our reality.

Another aspect of intention is that everything in the universe is somehow connected. This is true even though we cannot see this connection. The all-things-are-connected principle is embodied in Sir Isaac Newton's law of dynamics, and as part of modern astrophysics, researchers have amassed evidence of a universal energy field.

When we harness intention, dreams can become reality. Obey the following principles when creating a mental intention of healing:

1. **Become clear about your health objective.** Do you want to heal a part of your body? Do you want a particular illness to resolve itself? Whatever your desire, intention can accelerate the results. The more clarity you have about that desire, the better.

2. **Connect with your objective.** Realise that you are not separate from your objective. Imagine and experience yourself achieving

your health objective now. How do you look? How do you feel? The more fully you associate with your intention, the better.

3. **Believe in your objective.** What the mind believes the body achieves. Our thoughts shape our reality. A famous psychology experiment was carried out with a basketball team. A group of players were divided into two teams of equal ability. One team trained for an hour practising free throws, whilst the other team simply relaxed and visualised scoring from free throws. When it came to the test, and the teams had to take free throws, the team that simply visualised fared considerably better than the team that actually practised. Why is this? It is because they didn't miss any shots in their visualisations and therefore in their minds they actually had a stronger belief that they would score.

   Remember that the mind creates self-fulfilling realities. If you are convinced that no therapy will help you recover from your illness, you might be correct, but no more correct than the person who fully believes that he will make a full recovery from the so-called 'incurable' disease and then does. Whether you believe you will become completely healthy or not, you will probably be right. Make sure you believe.

4. **Let destiny work.** Once you have set an objective, allow destiny to take over and place your trust and faith in it. When you put a cake in the oven, you hand control of the outcome to fate. In the same way, trust in the process, knowing that the universal consciousness is working for you. Allow your objective to unfold in its own perfect manner without restricting it to a timeline. Don't be surprised if the outcome is better than you imagined.

5. **Accept all possibilities of your objective.** Ask yourself, 'How deserving do I feel of achieving my objective?' Some people unconsciously may feel undeserving of their intentions and have instinctively repelled their desires. Remove all such blocks to your healing objective by recognising that you are indeed

deserving and expand your ability to receive. If receiving this intention disrupts aspects of your life, recognise that the power of divine consciousness will work to address these issues also. Create space for your desire and allow it come into your life.

Most people are unaware of the hidden potential of their sub-conscious mind. We all have a store of powerful intelligence, which when tapped into can turn limitless aspirations into reality. We all have the ability to tap into this power, and one of the best ways to harness the healing power of your subconscious mind is to think *beyond* your health recovery: actively make plans for things that you are going to do after you have completely recovered your health. Remember again, where your mind goes your body follows.

Thinking Beyond Being Healthy Again

So, what are you going to do when you are completely healthy?

To begin this exercise, sit comfortably and relax. Take some time to ponder the question 'What do I really want from life?' What pleasur-able life aspirations do you have? What are your goals and dreams? Put your illness to one side and think about one thing that you want to experience or achieve. Choose a goal that you are in control of and that has no dependency on anyone else. Creating goals is about *you* and not what others want from you. Put aside what your family and friends think you should be planning, and decide on what you *really* want from the heart!

Now that you have chosen your goal, close your eyes and see yourself involved in that experience. Exercise all of your senses and imagine seeing what you will see, hearing what you will hear, feeling what you will feel. Are there any tastes or smells? Experience this future as if looking through your own eyes, making sure that the image is bright, colourful, vivid and distinct. As the image gets brighter, allow the physical sensation in your body to intensify. I'm sure that such a pleasurable experience merits a smile, so allow a broad grin to come to your face. When you feel like you have really captured the experience in your mind, allow your eyes to open.

Now that your eyes are open I want you to ask yourself, 'What is the first thing I need to do in order to realise this experience?' Is there a phone call you need to make? A place you need to visit? Some research you need to do? If so, do it now!

Immune Conditioning – the Powerful Healing Effect of a Positive Mind

Before we look at how we use our mind to enhance our immune system's ability to fight disease, let's look at how the immune system works.

The function of our immune system is to protect us from foreign micro-organisms such as viruses, bacteria, fungi and parasites. The immune system uses different strategies to neutralise these invaders. The first line of defence is the creation of a barrier; for example, the skin produces antibacterial substances, the nose secretes mucus, the mouth produces saliva, and the eyes release tears. If foreign organisms succeed in entering the body, they can then be expelled by specific mechanisms, such as sneezing or coughing for example, or destroyed by the cells of the immune system before they multiply and cause infection. Diseases occur when the immune system does not function properly.

We can imagine our body is like a sacred temple. This temple is surrounded by a wall – our skin – which helps to keep out potential invaders. This temple needs a good guard system to keep us safe from invaders who may try to sneak in and damage valuable treasure. (In our case, our health is the thing that is at risk.)

When intruders enter our body in the form of bacteria, virus or parasites, some will be escorted to a 'holding centre' to be examined, so that the correct 'special forces' can be sent out. These holding centres are called lymph nodes and are positioned in various parts of the body, such as the armpits, the groin, the neck, the gut, the abdomen and the chest. They help the body to get rid of foreign micro-organisms. When there is an immune response triggered by the presence of invaders, these nodes swell.

As children, a small organ called the thymus – which is situated in the chest between the breastbone and the heart – produces

T-cells. By the age of about ten all the T-cells should have been trained to find almost every bug, virus, microbe, bacteria and parasite that exists. The T-cells are special defenders that are tasked with searching and destroying infected cells. The T-cells move around our body in the bloodstream, finding good and bad cells. If a good cell is caught, it is checked before being released, but if an invader is found, a chemical signal is sent by special manager cells known as T4-cells to alert our defences of the invasion. Special T8-cells then respond to destroy the invader. When they come into contact with another cell that they now recognise as an antigen, they bind to it and destroy it. An antigen is the chemical part of the germ, cell or virus that your body recognises as not belonging. These T8-cells are needed to kill certain tumour cells, viral-infected cells and sometimes parasites.

There are also natural killer (NK) cells. Like T8-cells, they kill on contact, but the difference between them is that NK cells attack without first having to recognise the antigens, hence their name.

The remnants of the intruders are then removed by the macro-phages to the lymph nodes, so that they can do no further damage, before they are finally cleared away.

When the invasion is completely defeated, a suppressor T-cell sends out a second message to all the guards – the T-cells and the macrophages – to stop. If they were allowed to continue un-checked, too many good cells would be damaged.

At this point a second wave of guards arrives, and the T4-cells send for the long-term defenders, the B-cells. The B-cells learn to identify the intruder and produce millions of little poisoned darts. These darts contain strong chemical markers called antibodies, and from now on, if the temple is ever invaded by the same intruders again, a rapid response will recognise the intruder and defeat it.

Boosting Immunity Through Guided Imagery

Now that we know how the immune system works, wouldn't it be wonderful if you could train it to ward off illness? Well, the good news is that you can. The following visualisation technique has been used to bolster immunity, and evidence has shown that it can be used to modify the numbers of circulating white blood cells and natural-killer-cell activity, as well as other aspects of immune function. When researchers at the University of Aarhus asked volunteers to use similar guided-imagery techniques to boost immune-system efficiency, a study showed that there was a significant boost in natural-killer-cell activity over a ten-day period.

Immunity-enhancing Visualisation

1. With your eyes closed, visualise your immune system in a simple manner, perhaps based on the description earlier in this chapter: you might see an army of white guard cells, strong, alert and ready to protect your body.
2. Now imagine going right inside your body to the specific area you wish to heal. Notice what the area looks like. Perhaps you might see an infection or a diseased pool of black cells.
3. Now, with strong intention, see the powerful white cells encapsulating, overpowering and cleaning out these tiny black cells.
4. When all of the little black cells have been removed, notice the white cells realigning and continuing to patrol your body, ready to ward off any other invaders.
5. Now see a healthy vision of yourself standing confidently in front of you. See in vivid detail just how this healthy you moves, breathes and exudes health.
6. Finally, imagine stepping inside this healthier you, just as if you were fitting on a new suit. Take a deep breath in as you open your eyes. Notice how much better you feel.

The Mind–Body Link

The modern medical science of psychoneuroimmunology is confirming what many learned oriental doctors have known for centuries – that there is a direct link between the mind, the body and health. Science has revealed that the immune system can learn to respond to psychological stimuli such as a conversation, a news report, a smell or a taste. Actual biochemical changes take place in our bodies as a result of what is happening in our minds. Immune conditioning therefore works in much the same way as behavioural conditioning, which was made famous by the work of Russian scientist Ivan Pavlov.

Pavlov won a Nobel Prize in 1904 for his work on the role of enzymes and the control of salivation. He is remembered for his experiment showing that if a bell is rung whenever food is shown to a dog, in due course the dog will begin to salivate when the bell is rung without the food being present.

Animals, including humans, respond to many different kinds of stimuli. Unconditioned reflexes can be triggered by any sensory stimulus, such as colour, light and sound. For example, if a bright beam of light hits our eyes, our pupils shrink in response to the stimulus. Similarly, if a doctor taps below the kneecap, your leg swings out. These are built-in reflexes and are therefore 'unconditioned'. The body will respond in the same way every time this stimulus is applied.

What Pavlov discovered, however, was that environmental events that had absolutely no relation to a given reflex (such as a bell sound) could also, through practice, trigger a reflex (salivation). This learned response is what we call a 'conditioned' reflex. The process whereby we learn to connect a stimulus to a reflex is called conditioning.

Two eminent scientists, psychologist Robert Ader and immunologist Nicholas Cohen, discovered a very exciting application of Pavlov's experiments. In pioneering research, they found that we can pair a neutral stimulus, such as a taste, with a stimulus that alters immune-system function. Once conditioning has taken place, we can reproduce the altering effect on the immune system simply by introducing that taste.

In a recent experiment, German researchers injected volunteers with adrenaline, which elicits a temporary increase in natural-killer-cell activity. As the injections were administered, the volunteers were given sherbet. Through conditioning, the sherbet was capable of eliciting the same increase in natural-killer-cell activity as the adrenaline medication.

Immune conditioning has been proven to do more than modify immune function, and a host of studies have shown that it also produces measurable changes to our health. Experiments have shown that immune conditioning can alter the progress of arthritis, lupus, cancer and many other diseases.

Working at the University of Rochester, Robert Ader assisted in treating a young girl who had developed a severe form of systemic lupus erythematosis (SLE). The girl was suffering from high blood pressure, kidney damage and bleeding as a result of her condition. As part of her treatment, her doctors needed to use a powerful drug called cyclophosphamide to alter her immune response.

For three months each time the girl received the drug a perfume was released in the treatment room. During the months that followed the drug dosage was decreased but the perfume was continuously released during treatment sessions. The response was excellent: her lupus went into remission using only half the normal dosage of the medication.

The Healing Code Immuno-conditioning Programme

When practised diligently, this series of exercises will condition your immune response to greatly enhance your powers of recovery. They will allow you to harness at will the powerful healing potential of proven healing forces. You will link or anchor a selected food with activities that boost immunity, fight disease and enhance health and well-being. Through conditioning, you then snack on that food and without any conscious effort draw upon your own powerful healing potential.

Preparation for Immuno-conditioning Exercises

Step One – Choose Your Healing Food

In preparation, you will need to choose *one* food from the list below. Preferably choose a food that you like but have not consumed to any great extent. You must make sure that you can get this food all year round, or at least until you have completely recovered your health. The food choices are apples, dried apricots, grapes, prunes, oranges, raisins, strawberries and tangerines. This chosen food will become a staple of your diet and the snack food that you will eat regularly throughout the day.

Step Two – Choose Your Healing Word

In addition to the food, you will need a healing word, which you will repeat to yourself when eating the food, thereby triggering the healing anchor. You should choose a word that represents your intent, such as 'health', 'salud' or 'sláinte', the Spanish and Gaelic words for 'health'. Now let's harness the power!

Laughter Therapy

> *'He who laughs, lasts.'* – Mary Pettibone Poole

We often hear the old adage 'Laughter is the best medicine.' In 1979 Dr Norman Cousins decided to test this idea when he used laughter as a treatment for the spinal disease ankylosing spondylitis. Dr Cousins spent his career researching the role of laughter on health, and he, as well as others, went on to establish a whole host of benefits associated with laughter. These include:

- **Boosting immunity:** a number of studies, including one in 1994 led by H. M. Lefcourt, have established that laughter increases the count of natural killer cells and also raises the levels of antibodies and T-cells. Natural killer cells and T-cells are types of defence cells that attack foreign material in our bodies. Antibodies are our defence against disease. A 1985 study by Dillon, Baker and Minchoff found that after laughter there is an increase in antibodies (immunoglobulin A) in the mucus of the nose and respiratory passages. This has a protective capacity against many viruses, bacteria and other micro-organisms. The effect of laughter on our immune system is considered to be very significant with regard to many diseases including AIDS and cancer.

- **Pain relief:** laughter relieves pain through triggering the release of endorphins, which are the brain's natural painkillers. They induce a general sense of well-being when released.
- **Relieving stress:** laughter counteracts the harmful effects of stress. It is one of the most powerful anti-stress measures as it reduces the levels of the hormones of the 'fight or flight response', epineprine and cortisol. Laughter acts as one of the best muscle relaxants. It expands blood vessels and sends more blood to the extremities and muscles. Experiments have established that laughter significantly lowers high blood pressure by reducing the release of stress-related hormones and inducing relaxation. It also increases the release of adrenaline from the adrenal glands due to stimulation of the hypothalamus, which again causes relaxation. Laughter is akin to meditation, in that relaxation is an outcome. However, laughter is easier to do, and it is something we already do naturally.
- **Protection from heart disease:** laughter improves the blood circulation and oxygen supply to the heart muscles, significantly reducing the chances of blood clotting. It also provides an internal 'massage' of the organs, which stimulates digestion.

The Healing Code Laughter Exercise

For this stage you will need to hire your favourite funny film or stand-up comedy on video or DVD. Choose something that is guaranteed to give you lots of belly laughs. Sit comfortably with your chosen healing food close to hand. Leave the healing food alone and focus your attention only on the video. At your first big laugh say your healing word and eat your healing food.

Repeat this throughout the video, making sure *only* to consume the healing food right after laughing. Continue the exercise until all the healing food is consumed or the video is finished.

Repeat this exercise with a different comedy video each day for five successive days. After the fifth day continue the exercise frequently over the next three months.

Love Therapy

A number of clinical studies since the 1970s have confirmed that supportive human relationships have genuine healing properties. Research has established a link between social connection and reduced incidence of disease and increased life expectancy. A large-scale study based on 5,000 inhabitants of Alameda County, California, revealed that those individuals who enjoyed social interaction benefited from a dramatic increase in life expectancy. This study, which lasted 17 years, established that social connection and interaction provided protection against all types of cancer, dramatically lowering the risk of heart disease, and for those who did encounter illness, it significantly improved recovery rates. This is why attending support groups can considerably improve your health after illness.

A series of studies carried out by Janice Kiecolt-Glaser at the University of Ohio State established strong links between social interaction and strengthened immune function. Subjects with loving relationships had greater levels of natural killer cells, more responsive T-lymphocytes, stronger immune control over viruses and lower cortisol (the stress hormone) levels.

A fascinating series of studies conducted by Dr David C. McClelland have shown how the power of love and relationships affects our immunity. A group of student volunteers was asked to view a film about Mother Teresa. This video was specially designed to induce a positive, caring and loving emotional state. Those students who watched the movie of Mother Teresa had a significant increase in salivary immunoglobulin A, the protective antibody against viruses. Love, care and compassion have a positive impact on the immune system of the giver.

Studies at the Pittsburgh Cancer Institute showed that women with breast cancer had much higher levels of natural-killer-cell activity when they benefited from loving relationships. A further study at the University of Stanford found that women with advanced breast cancer saw dramatic improvements in remission when social interaction increased. These are particularly important studies as they show that natural killer cells can play a significant role in preventing the spread of cancer. We all know that babies need lots of love, human touch and nurturing to thrive. The same applies to adults, and science has now proven that love actually does heal.

Dr Dean Ornish, who has written numerous books on heart health, had this to say about love and health:

> Although there is more scientific evidence now than ever demonstrating how simple changes in diet and lifestyle may cause substantial improvements in health and well-being, one of the most powerful interventions – and often the most meaningful for me and for the people with whom I work, both colleagues and patients – is the healing power of love and intimacy and the emotional and spiritual transformation that often result from these. These include:
>
> • Rediscovering inner sources of peace, joy and well-being.
> • Learning how to communicate in ways that enhance intimacy with loved ones.
> • Creating a healthy community of friends and family.
> • Developing more compassion and empathy for both yourself and others.
> • Experiencing directly the transcendent interconnectedness of life.

So now we know that love is a powerful healer, let's harness this power fully.

The Healing Code Love Exercise

Step One

I want you to sit comfortably in a chair. Again, have your chosen healing food close to hand. This time I want you to recall a time when you felt completely loved and in love. Relationships can have good and bad times, but for this exercise you must only focus on the wonderfully positive moments that brought purely good feelings. Close your eyes and remember vividly a particular experience. Recall who was there, where you were, the sights, sounds, colours, smells. Importantly, feel the same physical feeling you had inside you.

When you are feeling the experience to its maximum, increase that feeling. Make the colours more vivid and bright, the sounds louder, and feel the physical sensation more strongly. Allow the waves of loving pleasure to swell over your body. Now that this feeling is again all-consuming, reach to your chosen healing food, say your healing word and savour the taste of the food in your mouth. Continue this exercise, reliving distinct moments or the same moment, over and over again for ten repetitions. Make sure only to eat the food when you clearly feel the sensations of love in your body.

Repeat this exercise every day for the next three months.

Step Two

For this exercise you will have the assistance of a partner, someone you care about and who cares about you.

Again have your chosen food to hand. Give and receive the biggest, most genuinely loving hug you can. When you can feel waves of compassion over your body, say your healing word and consume your healing food.

Repeat for ten repetitions every day for five days and frequently over the next three months.

Music Therapy

'He who sings frightens away all his ills.' – Anonymous

Music has been used as a healing ritual for thousands of years by many civilisations throughout the world. Recently there's been an increased interest in the healing benefits of music and how such activities can be used therapeutically in the medical setting. Scientific evidence has now established that music can be truly beneficial from a biological perspective.

There is considerable rationale to support the use of music to enhance immunity. Music's ability to alter mood has long been known, but more recently it has been scientifically established that music can alter autonomic-nervous-system (ANS) activity. The ANS, in turn, can modulate virtually every aspect of our immune function.

In addition to its significant immuno-enhancing effects, music can reduce the levels of the stress hormone cortisol, improve autonomic balance and increase positive emotion in both healthy populations and in individuals with a variety of conditions.

There seems to be an increased therapeutic effect when subjects not only listen to music but interact with it by dancing or drumming. In a study of drumming conducted by neurologist Barry Bittman, MD, it was discovered that a significant increase in natural-killer-cell activity took place when subjects drummed along to music. As we know, natural killer cells are an important component of our defences against cancer and other serious 'invasions'. The drummers also improved their ratios of dehydroepiandrosterone (DHEA) to cortisol, which further indicates an improvement in immune function. Group drumming in normal subjects enhances the activity of specific cellular immune components that are responsible for seeking out and destroying cancer cells and viruses.

The Healing Code Music Exercise

For this exercise you must interact with music in one of three ways. You can dance to the music (with or without a partner), you can sing along, or you can drum to the music. Select a music CD to play. Make sure that the music is 'positive' and suggests well-being.

When the music is playing, get in time, and when you feel that you are completely in harmony and joyously lost in the music, say your healing word and eat your healing food.

Repeat this ten times for the next five days and continue frequently over the next three months.

Prayer Therapy

People of religious faith have been shown in numerous studies to have advantages when it comes to health recovery. Religion and medicine have been closely interconnected within most cultures throughout most of recorded human history. In this modern era any link between prayer, religion and health may seem far-fetched for some people. However, recent studies have confirmed what many 'believers' suspected all along: there is a very significant biochemically measurable benefit to prayer and religious involvement. In a study performed by Harold Koenig, Harvey Cohen and Linda George at the University of Duke in 1997, interleukin-6 (IL-6) serum levels were measured in 1,718 participants. Subjects who attended religious services were 49% less likely to have high serum levels. High IL-6 levels are a biomarker of inflammation and are often found to be elevated in conditions such as diabetes, heart disease and cancer.

A further study conducted by M. D. Schaal at the University of Stanford in 1998 examined the relationship between religious involvement and immune function in 112 women with metastatic breast cancer. The study revealed a significant correlation between religious and spiritual expression and natural-killer-cell and T-cell counts. This again indicates that religious expression has a powerful influence on immune functioning.

As Koenig and Cohen say in their book, *The Link Between Religion and Health*, 'These are exciting times, for we stand at the brink of new discoveries that may unveil explanations for the religion–health relationship – ultimately providing clues that may empower us all and improve public health.'

The Healing Code Prayer Exercise

Practise this exercise through your own religious faith. If you are not a person who follows any religion or who believes in God, there is still no reason to overlook this exercise. You can simply perform the exercise by calling upon your own higher consciousness. When practising this exercise, you should find a time when you can be alone and undisturbed.

Place your healing food directly in front of you and, with intense focus, concentrate on the specific healing wish that you want embodied in the food. Visualise with such passion that you see the healing manifestation taking place in your head, as if it were already a reality. Now hold your hands over the food and close your eyes. Visualise divine healing energy coming through your body and flowing into your healing food from your hands.

If you wish, you may pray to God at this point, again calling for divine assistance with your healing wish. Now say the healing word and eat your healing food slowly but consciously, with a sense of inner conviction that your healing wish is actually passing through your entire body, through every cell, tissue and fibre.

Repeat this exercise 20 times over the next 10 days and continue each day for the next 3 months.

Practice Makes You Perfect

Repetition is a key factor in the success of the Healing Code Immuno-conditioning Programme. As we repeatedly practise the exercises, we create a neural pathway in the brain which is reinforced with each repetition. It is this repetition that creates the conditioned response that allows your subconscious mind to deliver firstly a greater sense of well-being and secondly an actual state of improved health.

Perform these exercises every day and before long you will start to feel better in yourself and improve the way you feel about yourself. Each time you perform these exercises recognise that you are moving closer to your health-recovery goal. The more you perform the exercises, the more likely it is that the recovery will happen sooner than you ever imagined.

The Healing Ritual and the Power of Dreams

You will remember that at the start of this chapter I described the way I responded when I was first diagnosed. I concentrated all my efforts on finding out everything that I could about MS; I found many books about the illness, which detailed all the potential difficulties I could encounter in grim detail. I became preoccupied with checking myself against each potential symptom and developed an unhelpful morning ritual in which I would check the strength of my legs, the quality of my vision, bladder function, etc. I convinced myself that each of these functions was worsening, and as a result my body started to follow. This was a particularly difficult phase for me, and I soon realised that these thought patterns were totally counterproductive to my recovery. Whenever you encounter yourself experiencing negative thoughts about yourself or your health, no matter how justifiable it might seem, you must use the techniques described in this chapter to reframe those thoughts into positive intentions.

Now that we understand the power of the subconscious mind, we understand that I was using my mind to manifest illness in my body, which was particularly unhelpful to my health recovery. I therefore had to create a new morning and evening ritual that would *assist* my subconscious to heal my body. To do this, I harnessed the power of dreams.

At night, when we sleep, our subconscious mind works most effectively and intensely. At this time the activity of normal consciousness is suspended, and when we enter into the sleep state, the activity of the subconscious takes over. Therefore, an optimum time for the acceptance of any autosuggestive formula is at night, when you lie in bed tired and are ready to fall asleep, or in the morning, when you are still in that half-awake state. Knowing this, you will never again allow yourself to fall asleep with thoughts of grief, sorrow, anger, guilt or any negative emotion, as this will influence the subconscious unfavourably. Always fall asleep with peaceful thoughts of health and happiness.

The Healing Code Power of Dreams Exercise – Doorway to the Subconscious

For this exercise it is useful to have a chain with 40 beads. You may also use a string with 40 knots tied in it. This will serve as an aid for autosuggestion so you don't have to involve the conscious mind in counting when you repeat the suggestion formula.

First of all, formulate the health wish you want to achieve in a short sentence *in the present tense* and in the positive form of a fact. For example, 'I am a non-smoker' or 'I am healthy.' By stating the fact in the present tense, your subconscious does not have the opportunity to mischievously place obstacles in the way of your wishes, as it would had the fact been stated in the future tense. Therefore, avoid phrases like 'I will stop smoking' or 'I will be healthy again.'

1. Just as you are about to fall asleep, take the string of beads and, with strong intention, whisper your health wish in a low voice or just in your thoughts, whichever is more comfortable for you. As you repeat your sentence, move your fingers from bead to bead. When you have reached the end of the beads you know that you have repeated the sentence 40 times.

2. Now relax and recall a time when you were extremely happy, confident and with a great sense of health and well-being. Let your mind recreate the sensations associated with that experience – the sights, sounds, colours, smells and, most importantly, the feelings within your body associated with that memory.

3. Next, imagine a flowing stream of bright white light entering your body at the centre of your chest – your heart. Allow this light to feed the existing sensation of joy, growing it stronger and stronger. Let this feeling develop until it fills your entire body and imagine it bathing you in bright white energy – allowing a broad smile to appear on your face. As you finish the exercise, again say the health wish.

You can use this exercise to programme numerous autosuggestions apart from good health. You can change unhelpful character traits, eliminate or promote behaviours and even develop artistic abilities. When you have witnessed the power of this exercise first-hand, you will use it to create many powerful influences for years to come.

In Summary

• You have learned some powerful new ways to run your own brain. When you consistently practise all of these exercises, you will alter the software in your head and manifest powerful benefits and changes to the way you feel very quickly. By embracing these techniques, you will not only benefit your health, but also significantly enhance the quality of your life and the lives of the people around you.

- For the next 12 weeks indulge yourself in consistent mental positivity. Continue to work through this book, but also spend time each day working on the mind-programming exercises in this chapter. You have already been called upon to perform exercises that will have created the mental foundation for your complete health recovery.

- Some of the exercises you need perform only once. For example, you only write your health recovery story once and produce one well-formed outcome. Other techniques, such as the Three Steps to Reprogramme Your Mind for Healing and Breaking the Curse, you will practise for the next couple of weeks and come back to them later as and when you wish.

- Integrate the Healing Code Immuno-conditioning Programme into your life for the next 12 weeks and beyond. You now have permission to enjoy time spent on an exercise that recognises the value of laughter, love, joyous music and sacred power. Take it as a gift.

- Make sure that each night before you enter into a restful night's sleep you perform the Healing Code Power of Dreams Exercise. Much of your body's self-healing happens when you are asleep, and this helps to maximise your healing potential.

If you encounter a day when you need motivation, why not harness Newton's law of motion? Newton's first law of motion states that an object at rest will remain at rest, and an object in motion will remain in motion. Once you get started, it is easier to keep going and make progress. After the decision has been made, one tiny first step gives you the momentum to keep going.

On such a day when you do not feel inclined to perform these mind-programming exercises, simply make this deal with yourself: decide to perform the exercise for just ten minutes right away. That is all. If after ten minutes you still do not feel like continuing, then you can stop – but only if you want to. This works like a dream. Once momentum is created, you never want to stop after just ten minutes. You can apply this motivation technique to all other elements of this book.

Perhaps one of the most important lessons of this chapter is that *you* are responsible for the way your mind operates. If you don't embrace this responsibility, somebody else will, and whether or not they will serve your best interests is a potential lottery. From now on it's your choice. *You* are in control.

So, we have looked in detail at the mind in our head. But the really wise among us realise that our mind permeates our entire being. Indeed, the ancients of the East understood that it is the mind stored within our bodies that has a profound effect on our state of health. The forces that intensely influence this bodily mind are called the emotions. Now let us look at how we can use our emotions to further enhance our return to health.

CHAPTER THREE

Step Two: Taking Charge of Your Emotions

E motional trauma and suppression affect our bodies. Consequently, emotional release acts to unlock our healing potential. Most ancient traditional systems of medicine, such as Chinese
medicine, place emotion at the core of illness. Some of the latest
scientific evidence supports many of these ancient Chinese medical
theories of the mind–body connection.

When I first heard that Chinese medicine linked particular
emotions with distinct organs in our bodies and with distinct
illnesses, I must admit that I thought it was far-fetched. How could
a single emotion affect a particular organ in your body in a precise
way? On closer observation, it became clear to me that the insight
was in fact very profound indeed.

Most Chinese medical theory comes from the simple observation of patterns in human behaviour. There are seven emotions
discussed in the ancient text *The Yellow Emperor's Classic of Internal
Medicine*. These are anger, fear, joy, sorrow, oppression, worry and
fright. Fear, for example, is associated with the kidneys and
bladder. The Chinese medics observed that before a battle commenced, warriors on both sides would always need to urinate. Now
let's apply this to the modern day. Have you noticed how the toilet
facilities on aeroplanes are in constant use, particularly by those
afraid of flying? Also, think about the last time you were called to
give a speech at short notice, or the last time you had to sit an
exam. Do you remember that you had to go to the bathroom first?

Chinese medicine sees a two-way association between emotions
and their linked physical organs. Therefore, severe or prolonged
dwelling on an emotion can cause problems with the associated

organs. Likewise, physical problems within an organ can cause difficulties with the associated emotion. The links between the emotions and the organs were all ascertained by simply observing the physical manifestations after strong emotions had been experienced or indeed suppressed: joy was linked with the heart, anger with the liver, sorrow with the lungs, worry with the spleen and fear with the kidneys.

The suppression of emotions such as anger, frustration and sorrow is seen as contributing towards many physical illnesses. When we suppress emotions with our conscious mind, we are essentially training our subconscious mind to accept these negative emotional feelings as normal. If this is done continuously, the subconscious mind will become confused and polarised. Negative life events will often start to seem acceptable and normal to the individual. In fact, a normal healthy emotional and physical state becomes almost abnormal, and this makes it more difficult to break out of the spiral of negative emotion and ill health. Take, for example, an unfulfilling or abusive relationship where the suffering party, rather than end the relationship, suppresses their emotions and convinces themselves that everything is fine. Even a physically and emotionally destructive relationship can continue for a long period of time, and when the relationship finally comes to an end, the injured party will often feel guilty and reject future nurturing relationships, gravitating instead towards an equally abusive relationship. The key to resolving such patterns is to retrain the subconscious mind to express negative emotions correctly.

In the clinic, this process is often aided by the release of suppressed emotions. This explains why clients will often experience an emotional release during or shortly after an acupuncture or healing session, often without knowing where this emotion came from.

Many people trap themselves in a chain of negative emotions. For example, if someone feels unreasonably frustrated or angry towards someone else, whether they express or repress this emotion, they will often feel very upset afterwards. This will often lead to feelings of guilt and low self-worth – ultimately they redirect this anger towards themselves. If this chaining of negative emotions happens continuously over time, it can often lead to severe anxiety or depression. So an initial negative emotion spirals into a whole series of lingering negative emotions – each one damaging to the person. The secret is to 'chain and spiral' positive emotions of confidence, self-worth and joy and in doing so help the client to release and ultimately extinguish the negative emotional feelings.

When it comes to treating illness, we often attempt to take the top layer off the symptoms without looking at the deeper emotional roots of the disease. If we don't treat the core emotional issue, symptoms may linger at a deeper level and manifest again with more illness. Then, when illness manifests, we may require more medication or more serious medical procedures, which in themselves cause even more emotional stress.

We are placing emotional suffering upon emotional suffering, and our body merely acts as an outward reflection of the emotion that resides inside. Are we exaggerating the significance of emotions? Well, according to the American Institute of Stress, up to 90% of all visits to general practitioners in the United States are a direct result of emotionally related disorders. Unfortunately, the treatment for emotional stress is usually fairly superficial medically speaking.

- A Harvard study found that men who worried about health, social conditions or finances had a significantly increased risk of coronary heart disease.
- A ten-year study reported in the *British Journal of Medical Psychology* showed that people who could manage emotional stress had a 40% lower death rate than people who could not handle emotional stress.

Where Is Emotion Held?

The leading research pioneer on psychoneuroimmunology, Dr Candace Pert, has said, 'In the beginning of my work, I matter-of-factly presumed that emotions were in the head or the brain. Now I would say they are really in the body.' This of course is true, and has been understood by Chinese medicine for thousands of years. A person experiences emotions in the form of chemical reactions in the body as well as the brain. The chemical reactions occur at the organ level, in the stomach, heart, liver, kidneys and muscles, as well as at a cellular level.

Chinese doctors discovered this link through simple observation. They also discovered that particular emotions are inclined to link with distinct organs, and consequently, strong emotions can manifest as problems with their related organs. We all encounter a variety of emotions in our daily lives. Some of these emotions manifest occasionally, while other emotions are so frequent they are seen as central to our personality. Some emotions are so prevalent that we don't even notice their presence and how they affect our relationships with people. But what exactly happens inside us when we experience emotions? How do our internal organs deal with the variety of them?

Emotional states are understood by modern medicine to bring about certain physical problems. For example, a long-standing depression can contribute to cardiovascular and immune-system disorders. When we face emotionally stressful situations, our brain releases biochemicals that help us to cope with the challenge and restore normal mood and behaviour. These chemicals, serotonin, noradrenaline and dopamine/endorphin, are often understood to have low rates in people prone to emotional disorders, such as anxiety and phobias, and those who are predisposed to overstress.

Modern life places a high degree of emotional turbulence at our doorsteps. How does mainstream medicine deal with emotion-related disorders? When it comes to these disorders, treatments are primarily controlling in nature, rather than aiming to address the underlying cause of the problem. By administering drugs that mimic the body's own chemical system, the emotional disorder is hoped to be brought under control. But the issue of dependency and side effects is a lingering one, and often the short-term benefits of medication do not translate into long-term happiness.

One of the key aspects of Chinese medicine is the holistic view of the human being. Chinese medicine understands that we are more than flesh and bones; we are also emotion and spirit. Behind the body's physical mechanisms there is an energetic blueprint. This concept is somewhat different from Western medicine. From Chinese medicine's point of view, emotion has the power to generate disease, just as a virus would. An emotional state can cause our chi, or life-force energy, to stagnate, flow in the wrong direction or drain away.

It is important to point out that all emotions are normal, and under normal circumstances they do not cause illness. They are part of who we are, and they contribute to our human nature. According to the great Taoist philosopher Zhuang Zi, 'We need emotions and feelings because how could we exist as individuals without them?' It is absolutely normal to experience a variety of emotions during your day: anger and frustration whilst travelling to work, worry about an exam or interview, sadness at someone's misfortune. It is virtually impossible to experience daily life without experiencing all of these emotions. Provided that they are transitory, they are of little significance to our health. However, whenever there is a predominance of one or more emotions, or when we endeavour to suppress one of these emotions, there can be consequences to our health that need to be addressed.

As we have seen, in Chinese medicine emotions when considered disease-causing agents can disturb the flow of chi and blood circulation, and damage the internal organs. On the other hand, the condition of the organs can directly affect our emotional state. For instance, fear can damage the kidneys and unhealthy kidneys can manifest externally through fear, thus creating a vicious circle.

According to ancient Chinese texts, 'Anger injures the Liver; Joy (excessive) injures the Heart; Grief and Sadness injure the Lungs; Worry injures the Spleen; and Fear injures the Kidneys.' Interestingly, all the emotions manifest themselves indirectly through the heart, which is the 'seat of the mind' in Chinese medicine.

How Emotion Causes Disease

Dr Candace Pert has discovered that the brain communicates with the cells of the immune system all over our body, and indeed, the immune-system cells communicate back to the brain using messenger cells called neuropeptides. In other words, if you experience anger, fear or worry, every immune cell throughout your body knows and interprets that emotion instantaneously.

So the brain and the cells throughout our body are in constant communication. These cells communicate throughout our bodies and also have a cellular memory. The emotion of fear, for example, produces more than fourteen hundred chemical reactions and activates more than thirty different hormones and neurotransmitters. The leading physiologist Dr Walter Cannon discovered in the 1920s that when a person felt that they were under extreme attack, the resultant emotion of fear would cause significant physiological changes in the body. A strong fear produced a signal that the body needed to defend itself or run away – what we call the 'fight or flight' response.

When a particularly stressful event occurs, the brain responds by triggering the release of powerful hormones from the adrenal gland, pituitary gland and the hypothalamus. The sympathetic nervous system, which is located throughout our body, is dramatically affected in a very real and rapid manner, and the repercussions are felt in every organ and tissue. Heart rate increases, blood pressure changes, we begin to sweat and so on.

It is perfectly normal for our bodies to react in this way. In fact, we are designed to react with the fight or flight response in order to protect us from potential danger. The problems occur when we make either of the following mistakes:

- We try to suppress the emotion and thereby ignore the natural fight or flight response.
- We dwell on the emotion and allow ourselves to linger in a constant fight or flight state.

So we get ill because we either repress our emotions or we get in a state of constant expression of emotion.

Learning From Children

To get an understanding of how we should react to emotional feelings, we only need to look at children. Young children have not been conditioned by the norms of society and will generally react to emotion in a manner that is truly natural. When they experience an emotion they express it freely, and then they move on from that emotion.

A young child who doesn't get what he wants will often have a tantrum. He'll throw himself on the ground and kick and scream. His anger will quickly transform into tears, but soon enough he will be watching *Barney* on television and giggling away happily.

An adult, on the other hand, who doesn't get the pay rise he had hoped for will often say nothing to the boss, yet internally be bursting with rage. He'll then go home holding on to that bitterness and struggle to sleep at night. Months or even years later he can still feel the bitterness at being let down by his employer.

Which approach to emotion do you think is better for your health? Of course it's the childlike approach of expression and then refusing to dwell on the emotion. The society norms of the world in which we live don't allow us to express our emotions with the freedom of a child. Nevertheless, there are ways round this.

As I mentioned earlier, this harbouring of old anger was something that I recognised as an issue I needed to overcome. As a teenager, I was dropped from the school's senior rugby team. Because I had scored three times for the team during the previous match, I felt that I had suffered a huge injustice. But instead of confronting the coach on the matter, I simply refused to play rugby for the school again so long as he was coach. Even though the coach himself asked me to play for the team again, I refused to even entertain the notion until he was no longer in charge. Teenagers can sometimes be naïve and often too principled for even their own good, but this was different: ten years later I would still spit bile when I recalled this story. I still harboured a huge amount of resentment towards this coach, even though common sense would tell you that it really wasn't a big deal. Holding on to this type of resentment was obviously a problem for me, but the root of the overall problem was the repression of these emotions when they were first experienced.

Emotional Repression

In certain cases we repress emotions automatically in order to deal with a situation that would otherwise be overwhelming. When we experience a loss, we will often move into a state of denial for a period of time until our emotions have a chance to catch up with the reality of the situation. Whilst this is generally considered normal, if emotions are repressed indefinitely this is almost always harmful. If we carry on as normal and pretend that all is well when it is not, then we are setting ourselves up for an even greater fall.

When we withhold feelings of anger, frustration, rejection or sadness, we build these emotions inside ourselves like a pressure cooker. The result is that we have inner anger, rage, sorrow and resentment, which we often redirect towards ourselves. Initially we learn as children to suppress our emotions consciously, but over time this becomes an unconscious act and powerful emotions can be blocked without any conscious effort. Look, for example, at the person who hates where he works. Years can pass without that person expressing his true feelings about his working environment.

The Strength of the Emotion

The stronger an emotion is, the more potential danger there is when it is repressed. Emotions that are trapped inside generally try to find a way to be expressed. This is the nature of emotion; it is meant to be expressed, and when we suppress it, the emotion just works harder to find expression. Often these repressed emotions will find unusual and unhealthy ways to vent themselves.

Emotions live on even if we try to cover them up. When anger and hostility are pent up over years, they can be set off easily, and when this is expressed, it can be quite ferocious. Often it will be a small thing that will become the straw that broke the camel's back, and the emotional backlash will seem above and beyond a normal response to the incident that unleashed it. When this finally happens, it is not unusual for similar outbursts to occur more frequently. Once the dam has burst, the emotion floods out more easily.

What Repressed Negative Emotions Do to Us

Repressed emotions, according to Chinese medicine, stop energy of "chi" flowing properly and cause it to stagnate in the body. The latest theories in biology suggest that repressed emotions have the real capability to create functional blockages in the neurology and the nervous system. Repressed emotions could therefore cause the brain to send the wrong messages to various organs in your body, with obvious consequences to your health. This means that emotions that have become trapped in your body, which you haven't let go of, can not only be a source of discomfort, but can also be a source of real physical problems.

The Journal of the American Medical Association has acknowledged that negative emotions can play a significant role in disease. In a 30-year study it was discovered that the major contributing factor to heart disease was anger. This recent study indicated that it's not working long hours, not stress, but rather it's the anger that causes heart attack. Furthermore, a Harvard Medical School study of heart-attack survivors found that the emotion of anger due to conflict doubled the risk of further heart attacks compared to those who remained calm.

We will usually do anything to get away from the strong feeling of a negative emotion. When you experience a deep sadness, for instance, you will try everything to escape that feeling, including sleep, immersing yourself in work and overexercising – anything to take your mind off the bad feelings. This is often the real reason why people drink too much, comfort-eat, abuse others, take drugs and much more. They do it because they want to get away from the harsh feelings of negative emotions.

The Subconscious Mind and Repressed Emotions

Repressed emotions are stored at the subconscious level. Again we must work through our subconscious mind to access and deal with these emotions. Your subconscious mind doesn't really want them, because they don't offer you any real benefits. Your subconscious mind wishes to serve you well, but the trouble is we don't often know how to access it properly. Once you gain access to your subconscious mind, it will assist you in dealing with these repressed negative emotions. The problem is that for many years you probably haven't asked it to do anything, and even if you have, you probably didn't ask it in a manner that would yield results.

Most of the time we simply communicate with our conscious mind, the part of our mind that we are aware of. But let's put it like this: your subconscious mind runs your body, your subconscious mind is in charge of your memories, your subconscious mind is in charge of your behaviour and your learning. It therefore makes sense that this is the part of your mind that you should be communicating with.

It is your subconscious mind that has the responsibility of releasing repressed negative emotions. In order to do this, the subconscious mind has to gain access to the emotional memories. Many people wonder why we need to care about something that happened to us in our past. Why do we need to let these feelings go? It's after all in the past, isn't it? And if it's in the past, surely that means that it's gone? Well, the truth is that if these emotions are lingering in your subconscious mind, it is almost as if it is being experienced to a degree each and every day. Let's take a simple test, again using the emotion of anger.

Remember something from your past that made you angry. Maybe it was a time when somebody you trusted completely let you down? As you think about it now, is there a feeling of anger associated with the memory? If you can still remember the anger as if it were happening in the present, then this is still locked in your subconscious memory and will potentially interfere with your current and future happiness. Why? Because if we live our lives with the additional burden of unresolved emotions from our past, there's less room to create a happy future.

As well as this, repressed negative emotions continuously send reminders in our lives of times when things weren't the way we wanted them to be. This obviously affects how we live our lives in the present.

This chapter addresses these repressed emotions and allows you to locate and clear these hurtful and harmful memories of the past. It consequently paves the way for emotional and physical healing to occur. My teacher, the world's leading hypnotherapist Dr Richard Bandler, was asked to describe the most mysterious healing experience he had encountered with a client. He told the story of a young woman who had experienced extreme brutality and abuse as a child. Her body still bore the marks from the beatings she had received from her father. Dr Bandler worked with the woman for some time, and when she had released the painful memories from her past, he noticed that something strange had happened. The marks and scars from her arms and body had completely disappeared. Dr Bandler asked the young woman what had happened to her scars to which she replied, 'What scars?'

Every time that you release a repressed negative emotion there is a healing effect. Obviously, not every healing effect will have such obvious external signs as with Dr Bandler's client, but nevertheless the healing effect will bring you forward mentally, emotionally and physically towards your goal of health recovery.

Before you can clear these repressed emotions, however, you need to identify them. To begin the process, you must access the memories and journal them. Once you have identified these emotional memories, you can then utilise the exercises in the remainder of this chapter to clear these emotions. These exercises address the main categories of repressed emotion. These include anger and frustration, guilt and loneliness, sorrow and grief, fear and, finally, worry. You can work through this entire process in quite a short space of time. However, the important thing is that you take the time to identify and address all the significant harmful emotional memories from your past by doing the following exercise.

Discovering Your Repressed Emotions

Step One – Identifying Dominant Emotions

Begin this exercise by considering which emotions play the most significant role in your life today. I am not necessarily talking about which emotion you express the most, but rather which emotion you feel the most. As you know, we often mask our emotions and the fact that we do this can cause these emotions to become repressed. So, from the following list, identify which are your dominant emotions. Which emotions provide the background soundtrack to your life at present?

- anger and frustration
- guilt and loneliness
- sorrow and grief
- fear
- worry.

Step Two – Recalling the Emotions of the Past

Once you have identified the most significant emotion in your current life, you are ready to move on to step Two. With pen and paper in hand, and making sure that you are warm and comfortable, allow your eyes to close. Become aware of the rise and fall of your breathing as allow yourself to relax. Now, focusing on your heart, imagine that you are breathing in and out of your physical heart. As you breathe, allow your thoughts to travel back to the last time that you encountered a strong feeling of that current significant emotion. As you recall that feeling, breathe deeply. That emotional feeling will either dissolve or it will remain. If the emotion remains, it can be deemed a repressed emotion that should be cleared.

When observing this emotion, recall who was there, what you heard and what was said, why you felt that emotion and the physical sensation you had in your body. If that emotion had a voice, what would it say to you? For example, 'I feel angry because this person violated me' or 'I feel sad because I lost this feeling of love.' At this point slowly open your eyes and record all of these details in a journal. Allow this memory to fade away and drift back into a state of relaxation. Now allow your mind to travel back to another previous encounter with a significant emotion from the list. It may be the same emotion again or it could be a different emotion. Once again journal the details of this memory before you allow it to fade away. Take your time and continue to work through this process until you have accessed and written down all the clear incidences of significant and strong emotions in your life, going right back as far as possible into your early childhood.

It is important to remember that as you are accessing your subconscious mind you should allow yourself to be completely relaxed. Remember that there are no time limits, and if distracting thoughts flow into your mind, simply observe them coming and going and soon enough your emotional memories will come to you without any conscious forcing or reasoning out what you think the memories ought to be.

Step Three – Beginning the Healing: Pulling Out the Pain

This powerful emotional-healing exercise releases many repressed negative emotions in general and paves the way for complete clearing using the remaining exercises in this chapter.

Part One – Locating Past Emotions

As you sit relaxed, allow your mind to recall a past emotional experience that was painful. Notice what you remember, who was there, what they were wearing, what you could hear. As the memory is retrieved, you will become aware of a change of physical sensation in your body. Take note of this area, as it is where the energy of this past emotional memory is stored. Allow the memory to fade away, letting the visual memory disappear into the distance.

When you work through different memories, you may notice that the location of the physical sensation changes as each emotional memory surfaces.

Part Two – Accessing Stored Emotions

Read through this part of the exercise three times or until you are familiar enough with the process to proceed from memory.

This stage of the exercise explores your subconscious feelings and allows you to reprogramme and create positive subconscious patterns. You will with practice gain access to many stored memories. More importantly, you will resolve the emotional trauma associated with these memories.

1. As you relax in the chair with your eyes closed, again bring your attention to the area where the past emotion was stored in Step One. Imagine opening a chamber of the past emotion and allowing the energy to release itself like steam from this area. Visualise allowing all the steam to release and gather into a grey cocoon shape on the left-hand side of your body.

2. Now imagine a ball of white energy gathering in the centre of your abdomen. Visualise energy from your brain gathering and descending down the centre of your body until it reaches the energy gathered at the centre of your chest. Allow these energies to combine and descend to the white energy gathered in the centre of your abdomen. Now imagine this energy forming a small version of yourself.

3. Visualise this energetic version of yourself slowly starting to ascend up the centre of your body until it leaves through the top of your head. As it leaves, notice it is still connected to your physical body through a silver energetic cord.

4. In your mind, see your energetic form floating over the energy cocoon on the left-hand side of your body. Notice within this grey cocoon cylinders of black energetic emotional clusters. These clusters are connected to the cocoon by energetic cords and represent the memories of painful emotions such as humiliation, rejection, shame and abandonment. Visualise your energetic self gathering these dark clusters, and now as you imagine connecting to a higher power, begin the process of understanding, forgiving and letting go of the emotional charges attached to these mem-

ories. Notice how these dark emotional clusters begin to pulsate and change colour from black to white.

5. At this point, focus on the energetic cloud and begin separating the hurtful memories from the wisdom and knowledge gathered from the experience. Imagine gathering this knowledge in the form of sparkling white energy and allow it to drift over to your right-hand side. The energy that remains gathered on your left-hand side represents the pain and hurt. Notice how it has formed into thicker, dark, black energy.

6. Focus on the right-hand side of the room, and again notice the bright, pure white energy. As you inhale, deeply visualise this energy being absorbed back into your physical body. Allow your body to feel empowered with each breath as it can now review these past experiences without any associated feelings of pain or hurt.

7. Next, focus on the dark, turbid energetic cloud on your left connected to the cocoon by an energetic cord. Now imagine an angelic figure descending from above and severing this energetic cord with a sword. This sword represents your decision to regain your power, as you are no longer willing to be burdened or repressed by painful memories. This act severs any last connection or attachment to toxic emotions. Visualise the dark cloud floating up out of the room, through the ceiling and out into space.

8. Now imagine waves of love and mercy descending towards earth from the higher power. As this wave of love and mercy touches the ascending dark cloud, it immediately explodes and transforms into blue crystal drops of divine healing energy. Visualise these drops pouring down like rain on your small energetic self. As you inhale, allow this energy to enter your physical body, feeling the divine healing light penetrate and radiate throughout your entire being.

9. Allow your small energetic self to re-enter the top of your head and travel down the centre core of your body, drawing the energy back into your lower abdomen. Finally, visualise reabsorbing the energetic cocoon back into your body and relax. After a few mo-

ments of quiescence, take a deep breath and allow your eyes to open.

Step Four – the Healing Code Emotional-clearing Programme

Next, starting with the first significant emotion you identified in Step One, turn to the section of the Healing Code Emotional-clearing Programme that relates to that emotion. Score the strength of feeling you currently have towards this memory on a scale of one to ten, with ten being a very strong, vivid and perhaps painful memory and one being a rather indistinct memory that doesn't bother you. Work through these exercises until this emotional memory is cleared or at least below two on the scale.

Continue through the process until you have addressed and cleared the strong, painful memories in the sequence as they occur in your journal, beginning with the most recent emotion. When you have worked back to as far as your earliest disturbing memory, you will have addressed these emotions and completed the exercise.

As you work through this exercise, memories may come flooding back that had long been forgotten. Like peeling the layers of an onion, as one emotional disturbance is cleared another one surfaces, which had until now been repressed. These emotional memories sometimes come flooding back during dreams, when your subconscious mind can communicate more freely. When this happens, journal this recently remembered experience and work through the relevant exercises again.

How the Pulling Out the Pain Exercise Works

Our present emotional life has been shaped by our perception of events that occurred in our past, often in the formative years. These experiences very often sink deep into our psyche and remain hidden from our consciousness through repression or denial. The Pulling Out the Pain Exercise is used to gain access to subconscious past emotional experiences. The goal of the exercise is to free yourself of these repressed emotions.

When first practising this exercise, you may find that you unconsciously choose memories that are not intensely painful, or that you find it difficult to access memories at all. As you practise, you will find that painful stored emotional memories will come to the surface. Memories will come to the surface when higher consciousness senses that the timing is right and you are ready to heal.

This shengong exercise, which literally means 'working with the mind', is divided into two stages. In the first stage you will locate where in your body past repressed emotions are stored. In the second stage we will access these stored emotions, release and heal them.

Begin the exercise by sitting comfortably in a chair, feet placed on the floor, hands resting on your lap. Breathe naturally and relax into yourself.

The Healing Code – Emotional-clearing Programme

Anger and Frustration

Generally speaking, anger is linked to the liver and gall bladder in Chinese medicine. When anger is prevalent, the energy, or chi, rises up, causing headaches and migraine, and can also attack the digestion, causing symptoms such as nausea, diarrhoea and conditions such as irritable bowel syndrome (IBS).

The following symptoms are frequently associated with anger's impact on the liver and gall bladder: indecisiveness, eye problems, headaches, muscle tension, feeling wound-up, depression, upset digestion, sour regurgitation, nausea, vomiting, tightness in the centre of the chest, pain under the ribcage, tiredness, dry skin, muscular weakness and spasms, dizziness, pins and needles, weak nails, waking up during the night, nightmares and period-related problems such as premenstrual tension.

The following conditions are frequently considered by Chinese medicine to have been influenced by anger: cerebral haemorrhage, stroke, cancer and heart attack.

The repression of anger is understood to cause chi to stagnate. When this happens over a long period of time, the anger turns to depression. Western psychology frequently interprets depression as anger turned inwards, and Chinese medicine concurs with this view. Chinese medicine will frequently see cancer as being caused by chi stagnation, and interestingly, strong recent scientific evidence has linked depression to the formation of various forms of cancer. Medical research has revealed that depression is associated with the poor repair of damaged DNA, which can be a precursor to cancer.

The process where abnormal damaged cells die and are flushed from the body is called apoptosis. Most of us develop abnormal cancer cells, but most of us do not develop cancer, because apoptosis causes those cells to be eliminated from the body just like any other toxin. Apoptosis is our body's key defence against cancer cells. As repressed anger can lead to depression, which in turn reduces natural-killer-cell activity, this makes it harder for the body to eliminate these abnormal cells. So naturally if we have been inclined to repress anger or have experienced depression, the expression or release of anger should help to restore balance and protect against various forms of cancer.

We saw earlier that Western medicine also recognises the impact anger can have on health. A report in the *American Journal of Cardiology* found that anger can seriously damage your health. A study showed that when people remembered an incident that made them angry, the pumping efficiency of the heart drops by on average 5%. A drop of just 7% is thought to be dangerous.

A further study at the University of Duke found that excessive anger was a higher predictor of mortality than smoking, high cholesterol and high blood pressure. Students at the medical school completed questionnaires and those with the highest scores for hostility and anger were a staggering 7 times more likely not to reach the age of 50 than those with lower scores.

Anger is controlled by sadness. This explains why children will get angry and after screaming they will quickly turn to tears. After this expression of sadness balance is restored. So the Chinese doctor will occasionally try to elicit sadness if the client is experiencing a constant state of anger.

Anger is an automatic response for many people. This often happens when people are frequently exposed to other angry people or an angry environment. Over time we are often unaware of what causes our anger and it just builds up. In this modern world we live in where the pace of life has increased, whilst the quality and quantity of leisure time has been steadily eroded, there has been an increase in anger, frustration and resentment and consequently an increase in the exposure to the associated conditions previously mentioned.

The Stolen Axe – a Taoist Tale From China by Lieh Tzu

A woodcutter went out one morning to cut some firewood and discovered that his favourite axe was missing. He couldn't find it anywhere. Then he noticed his neighbour's son standing near the woodshed. The woodcutter thought, 'Aha! That boy must have stolen my axe. I see how he lurks about the shed, shifting uneasily from foot to foot, greedy hands stuffed in his pockets, a guilty look on his face. I can't prove it, but he must have stolen my axe.'

A few days later the woodcutter was surprised and happy to come upon the axe under a pile of firewood. 'I remember now,' he said. 'It's just where I'd left it!'

The next time he saw his neighbour's son, the woodcutter looked intently at the boy, scrutinising him from head to toe. 'How odd,' he thought. 'Somehow this boy has lost his guilty look . . .'

'Holding anger is like grasping a hot coal with the intent of throwing it at someone else; all the while you are the one getting burned.'
– Buddha

Holding anger, bitterness and resentment is like creating a poison for someone and then taking it yourself every day. The American humorist Josh Billings was wise when he said, 'There is no revenge so complete as forgiveness.' What better way to triumph over someone who caused you harm, but for you to be unharmed?

We generally hold anger for reasons of self-preservation. If we hold such resentment, we mistakenly believe that this puts us on extra guard against the same harm being done to us again.

Releasing Anger Exercise

Step One – Awareness

Take a sheet of paper and write down a list of all the names of people against whom you still hold a significant grudge. Describe how they caused you harm and the consequent anger you now hold for them.

Step Two – Perspective

Close your eyes and one by one visualise becoming the person who caused you pain. Now as that person, ask yourself why you caused the hurt. Ask what your intentions were and about your underlying beliefs. Continue to ask the question until you receive an answer that you can accept as reasonable. The answer does not have to be acceptable as an excuse, just a reasonable explanation of why the incident took place. For example, someone who caused serious injury from a driving accident rarely sets out to cause any harm, so a reasonable explanation might be that they were distracted in some way whilst driving. No matter how horrific the incident, there is an explanation for it. Again, it does not mean that you condone the actions in any way; it just explains the possible reason why it happened.

Step Three – Forgiveness

Taking the original list, and having seen the incidents from the other person's perspective, close your eyes and notice how you feel about that person now. If you no longer harbour any resentment towards this person, mark them off your list, as you are now liberated from the harm that they caused.

If anger and resentment still linger, continue with the following exercise.

Completing Forgiveness

All of us have had things happen to us that have hurt us. We wish these things never happened, but they did. However, if we are still suffering as a result of these actions years later, it is because we have held on tightly to their memory. We are empowering the perpetrator of the harm by allowing the memory to linger on. We can't undo the incident. But we don't have to. At this point all we have is a stored memory of the incident and we are troubled not by the incident itself but rather by our memory of it. This is very different, because although we can't change the incident, we certainly can change our memory of it. Remember that we are not the sum of our experiences, but rather the sum of the perception of our experiences. Therefore by changing the memory, we in fact change who we are – forgiveness won't change the past, but it will enlarge the future.

Step One

Sit yourself down comfortably. Close your eyes and recall the person and the incident for which you still harbour a grudge. Notice the image you create. What is the size of the image? Are you within the incident and seeing the image again as you saw it when it happened? Is it moving or still? Is it coloured or black and white? What are the sounds and voices that you associate with the image?

Step Two

Now we are going to alter the memory. The process resembles the 'Breaking the Curse' exercise on page 45. Imagine the person who you held the grudge against having Mickey Mouse ears. When they speak they have a squeaky voice. Shrink them to half their normal size. Now drain the colour out of the picture entirely. Imagine there is silly music playing in the background – use *Chitty Chitty Bang Bang*. Now disassociate from the image and see it as a TV screen. Visualise turning the TV off and see the picture fading away into a white dot. Repeat this exercise until you no longer feel the same sense of anger towards the person.

'Forgiveness does not change the past, but it does enlarge the future.'
– Paul Boese, author

The NLP Forgiveness Technique

This method is a more thorough version of the Releasing Anger Exercise and is particularly useful if you are angry or resentful towards someone who has harmed you in the past but who is no longer part of your life.

The goal of this exercise is to resolve lingering anger and resentment. Forgiving others does not mean condoning the behaviour of the person who harmed you, or changing your own values that were violated. In fact, an important element of this exercise is to reaffirm your own values and to use them to choose ways of coping resourcefully. The inner strength that forgiveness brings you will make it easier to uphold your values and standards in the future.

Step One – Identifying Anger/Resentment

Identify the person and the event for which you still carry anger and resentment and would like to reach forgiveness and resolution. Notice how you feel about this person and score it on a scale of one to ten, with ten being extremely angry and one only slightly angry.

Step Two – Identifying Forgiveness

Next, identify an experience of forgiveness you have had. You can choose 1) someone you once resented but now when you think of that person it is only with feelings of forgiveness and compassion, or 2) someone who harmed you but you forgave them right away because you recognised that they had harmed you accidentally. For example, a small child could have hurt you but you would instantly forgive him because it was an accident and he was too young to recognise the consequences of his actions.

Step Three – Compare Approaches

Now compare the experiences in Steps One and Two and notice any differences that exist between these memories. Notice the location of the images when you recall them. Notice any differences in colour and brightness. Notice any differences in the sounds and the voices. Notice if you are in the middle of the event as it is happening or are disassociated and observing the images. Finally, notice the differences in the physical sensations you feel in your body.

Step Four – Address Any Objections

Now ask yourself if you carry any objection to reaching forgiveness with this person. The most common objections are of three types:

1. Forgiveness would seem to mean condoning the behaviour and violating your values and standards. However, forgiveness does not mean condoning the behaviour; it simply means refusing to be hurt by the behaviour for any longer than you have to – despite the behaviour. Your value system was violated, and at this point you can simply recognise that these values are still important to you.
2. Forgiveness might also mean that you appear weak. However, forgiveness is the ultimate sign of strength, and overcoming anger through forgiveness leads to even greater inner strength.
3. Forgiveness could remove protection from a repeat of the incident. This is valid, but simply having awareness satisfies this function without having to hold on to destructive resentment. At this point plan a possible future response. Could you educate the person who harmed you? How would you protect others from being harmed in the future?

Step Five – Altering Perspective

Now briefly observe the incident from different perspectives. First, imagine it from the view of a third party who might have witnessed the incident. Next, imagine stepping into the body of the person who harmed you. Do you learn anything new about this incident? Write down any additional information you get about how this person sees, hears and feels things.

Step Six – Switch Approaches

Now, one at a time, adjust your sensory memory of the anger/resentment experience so that you recall it in the manner you recalled the forgiveness experience. Shift the location of the images to where the forgiveness images are stored. Alter the colour and brightness so that it complies with the way in which you view the forgiveness images. Adjust the sounds and the voices to concur with the forgiveness model. Notice how the physical sensation in your body now changes and becomes more like the forgiveness model when you observe the anger/resentment experience through this new template. For example, if the forgiveness experience was bright and colourful whilst the anger/resentment experience was dark, change it so that the anger/resentment experience is bright and colourful.

Step Seven – Test

Now again think about the person you used to feel anger/resentment towards. Notice how you feel about that person now. Score the feeling yet again on a scale of one to ten and compare this to the score you observed at Step One. You will normally feel much more positive about the incident at this point. If not, go back over the process and make sure that you are mapping across the sensory approaches properly.

Beating the Bag Exercise

This is an ancient Chinese technique for safely releasing repressed anger. In the original form of the exercise a large rice bag would be used, but for our purposes we can use a large cushion or pillow.

1. Find a quiet place in your house where you won't be disturbed.
2. Place the cushion or pillow on the floor and kneel in front of it. Making fists with your hands, bring them down from above your head, beating on the cushion in a rhythmic movement.
3. Allow yourself to feel anger bubbling up to the surface, and if you recall any situations that made you feel particularly angry, allow them to be expressed as you beat on the cushions.

4. Now, in rhythm with the beating of the cushion, shout out the sound 'Gwow!' This is also used to release stagnant angry energy. Shout out the sound for about forty strikes and then change the word to 'No!' If you feel more anger coming up, feel free to use stronger language – that's why you are using a quiet place in your house.

5. Repeat this exercise for about ten minutes every day for ten days.

'To err is human, to forgive divine.' – Alexander Pope

Guilt and Loneliness

Chinese medicine associates the emotions of joy and love with the heart. The emotions of guilt and loneliness are also associated with the heart. The Chinese consider the heart the 'emperor organ' and it's seen as the 'supreme controller'. Its function is to keep the other organs functioning harmoniously, so when the heart is affected by emotions of guilt and loneliness, the person will often feel out of control and anxious. Chinese medics understand that the heart houses the 'shen', or the mind.

The latest medical science lends support to this ancient understanding of the heart. We now know that we do actually think with our hearts. The heart is our body's most important endocrine gland, and in response to our experiences, our heart produces and releases hormones that affect every operation in the limbic structure, what we know as our emotional brain. Sixty-five per cent of the cells in the heart are actually neural cells, identical to the cells found in the brain and operating through the same neurotransmitters that occur in the brain.

The heart is linked to every major organ in the body. Half of the heart's neural cells translate information sent from all over the body so that it can keep the body working as one harmonious whole. The other half of the heart's neural cells form a connection with our brain and carry a continuous dialogue between the brain in our heart and the brain in our head.

The following symptoms are frequently associated with an energetic imbalance in the heart, often caused by guilt, loneliness or excessive excitement: palpitations, anxiety attacks, insomnia, propensity to startle easily, daytime sweating, mania, restlessness and extreme confusion.

Two of the emotions seen as detrimental to the heart are guilt and loneliness. Many cultures around the world assocaite the heart with love and human connection. The emotions of guilt and loneliness are all about disconnection from friends, loved ones and society in general. Therefore addressing issues around guilt and being alone brings us towards repairing the emotional damage done to the heart.

All of us understand what it's like to feel guilty about something. Guilt makes us feel that we are unforgivable. Whilst this experience is common, it is also detrimental to our health. Feeling guilt causes a sense of anguish about a past action that cannot be changed. The purpose of this feeling is to ensure that you do not repeat the mistakes of the past. The problem, however, is that it does little to enable us to forgive ourselves, make amends for our mistakes and to move forward positively and free of emotional baggage from the past.

Guilt involves seeing your mistakes but not knowing what to do about them or else refusing to correct them. Guilt is therefore a negative, paralysing emotion. The problem with guilt is that it is often wrongly seen as a virtue. The Judaeo–Christian concept of 'original sin' – for which we personally are not responsible – firmly establishes the importance of guilt in our minds. We are born guilty. Furthermore, the presentations in several religious traditions can give us the impression that one should feel guilty or ashamed simply for having fun.

But whilst repentance is a very honourable attribute, guilt alone is generally a very negative force unless it leads us towards repentance. Dwelling on guilt simply creates the self-belief that you are evil and unworthy. It leads towards self-hatred and self-loathing.

The word 'guilt' stems from the same old English word as gold, 'gylt'. Originally when you had done something wrong, you made a payment in time or money and then by definition you were free of guilt. The problem with the guilt that we experience today is that it has become a permanent state of mind for some people. It has become a neurotic preoccupation, rather than a fair and proper assessment of a wrongdoing followed by action that leads to reparation.

Part of being human involves making mistakes and hurting other people. This is almost an unavoidable part of the human experience, and wallowing in guilt does not help you or anyone else. It will not do anything to prevent future harm or suffering either. Understanding this is the first step towards liberating yourself from guilt.

If you are holding on to guilt about something, the first thing that you need to do is show compassion for yourself. Whatever you did that you feel guilty about you did for a reason. The course of action you took may have been wrong, but as a human you make mistakes. Showing this compassion towards yourself is much more effective than guilt in helping you to determine the proper course of action that should have taken place. Once you show compassion for yourself, you can identify the steps you need to take to move towards reparation. This might mean making an apology, or may involve making some significant changes in your life. Understanding what this reparatory action is goes towards healing yourself as well as anyone that you may have hurt. Learn from your mistakes, but don't beat yourself up. Recognise that you are born good, love yourself and do your best. Recognise this and then you will realise that there is no place for guilt in your life.

Feeling guilty about an incident never makes it disappear. You can make changes in your life towards being a better person more effectively without feeling guilty about who you have been in the past.

If you are affected by guilt, then working through these five steps in the following exercise will free you from this harmful emotion.

Resolving Guilt

Step One – Understanding Responsibility

First of all, reflect on what it is you feel guilty about. Upon reflection, it may prove that it was not your responsibility or fault at all. Blaming yourself for everything negative that happens can in fact be a form of self-centred behaviour. Obviously, if you have been careless, thoughtless or intended to cause problems, then you should take responsibility and make sure that you will not repeat this regrettable action.

Task: write down the event that you feel guilty about and explain why you think you are responsible.

Step Two – Understanding Motivation

Any act done with positive intention cannot be seen as negative even if other people were harmed by it. True, we could have made mistakes because of poor communication or improper attention, but if this is the case, you must focus on improving this attribute rather than dwelling on the negative outcome.

Task: write down what circumstances outside of your positive intention caused the negative outcome.

Step Three – Change or Acceptance

If there is something you can do to change yourself or the situation, you should change it. If there isn't anything you can do to change yourself or the situation, then you simply must accept it and let it go.

Task: write down what you can do now to change the situation or to change yourself so that such a situation doesn't arise again. What is the first step you can take now to create this change? Is it a phone call? Is it going to see someone? Whatever it is, do it now! Not acting where we can leads to further frustration and further guilt in the long run.

Step Four – Analyse the Use of Feeling Guilty

If you have made a mistake, self-condemnation does little to remedy the situation. Remorse is constructive only when it calls you to react to make good any harm that was done. Based in the present, it is intelligently concerned with the future effects of your actions, and it leads to remedying the damage already done and to caution against repeating such an act.

Step Five – Forgiveness

Making mistakes is part of being human: if you don't make mistakes, you are definitely not living as a normal human being. Importantly, if you cannot forgive yourself, you will never be able to properly forgive others. This is not a good quality to have. Forgive yourself now and move forward without dwelling on the past.

Occasionally, it is too late for you to make reparations and you cannot go to the person and apologise or make good what wrong was done. If you feel guilty, it has to be because you hurt or neglected a person that you cared about. Importantly, this person is also likely to be someone that cared about you. If this person loved you, they would most likely forgive you. Therefore your inability to forgive yourself is not acting within the wishes of that person. You must honour that person now by forgiving yourself and carrying out a good deed – perhaps for someone you don't even know.

   Task: if it's possible, go to the person whom you harmed and, having carried out the task in Step Three, ask for their forgiveness. If you cannot ask this person for whatever reason, then write down your apology in detail in the form of a letter. When you are finished, burn the letter, sending your request for forgiveness into divine consciousness.

Defeating Loneliness With Social Connection

The importance of social connectedness was first established in the 1970s with a series of important research studies. Population studies in the USA and Europe during the same period measured the characteristics of social ties to evaluate possible relationships with disease and demonstrated that those with low social support and loose social ties risked earlier death. During the 1990s clinical studies in cardiovascular disease and cancer also confirmed the link between social connection and increased survival rates. Patients suffering a myocardial infarction appeared to have a higher than expected recovery rate if they had social support, lived with someone or were married. Women with breast cancer had lower mortality risk if they had a social network. Researchers have examined pathways by which social networks might influence health and have found strong emotional support was related to a higher recovery rate in the six months following a myocardial infarction. In Australia a study of patients with a range of cancer in an advanced stage lived longer if they had four or more people with whom they could share their feelings.

The temptation when recovering from a challenging illness is to become introspective and retreat into your shell. There is now strong evidence that this is the wrong thing to do. Now, more than at any other time, you should seek social support and connection. As part of increasing your social connection, make sure to include the following:

1. Spend time every day with friends and family.

2. Spend time connecting in social settings such as sporting events.

3. If you follow a faith, attend religious services.

4. Volunteer for charity work – reach out to others.

Sorrow and Grief

Chinese medicine primarily associates the emotion of sorrow with the lungs. Severe sorrow or grief affects both the lungs and the kidneys. The lungs govern breathing and respiration, which help to maintain sufficient levels of energy. The lungs also spread what is called the 'wei chi', or defensive energy, which defends us against illness. This is not dissimilar to the concept of the immune system. When the lungs are weak, this defensive energy is weak and we are more prone to illness. Recent studies have confirmed this to be true. In 1975, 52 people took part in a study. Half of the group had suffered bereavement and were tested two weeks and six weeks after they had suffered the loss. The immune systems of those who had lost someone were seriously suppressed, whilst the control group remained normal.

Some of the symptoms and illnesses associated with lung weakness are shortness of breath, a weak voice, asthma, bronchitis, daytime sweating, a tendency to catch colds or flu, coughing, tiredness, constipation and diarrhoea.

Sadness in response to losing a loved one is something that all of us experience at some time in our lives. Unresolved grief is often a factor in a wide range of conditions where immunity can be seriously affected.

Overcoming Sorrow – the Grief-resolution Process

People who are grieving or dwelling on sadness often mistakenly linger on thoughts about the ending of the relationship, rather than focusing on the loving relationship itself. Whatever you focus on brings back the emotion of that time and, with it, all the associated unpleasant feelings. Because the event was often traumatic, it is remembered in vivid detail and you can feel its full intensity.

When experiencing sadness or grief, it is for the loss of something that you felt was precious and special. Focusing on this unpleasant ending makes it impossible to experience the loving feelings that you had.

Step One

Make a list of everything that you loved and appreciated about the lost relationship.

Step Two

Many people get over their loss but often with a sense of resignation. When they think about the lost person, they would often sigh, shrug their shoulders and breathe shallowly. It is clear in this case that the grief has not been resolved fully. It was 'dealt with' only to the extent that it was repressed and controlled so that they could carry on.

There is, however, a more positive way of dealing with loss. When you can speak about the person with softness, care and happiness, and it draws out a smile, then you have dealt positively with the loss. When you can recall your loved one as if they are right there with you, and that makes you feel good, this kind of response is clearly more beneficial to you, as it provides you with access to all the enjoyable feelings that you had with the person that is now gone.

Think now about someone who is special to you in an existing relationship. Notice how you represent that person in your mind. What is the picture you create? Where is the person located? Are they on the left, right or right in front of you? Do you see them in colour or black and white? Are they life-size and three-dimensional? Do you see the person moving and breathing? What are the sounds and voices you hear in your head? What is the physical feeling you get in your body?

Now positively recalling a lost person should really be no different from recalling a person you love who is physically absent for a short time. This therefore becomes the model of how you should reprogramme your mind.

Step Three

Take a few moments to relax, with your eyes closed. Having recalled the person from your existing relationship, bring to mind the person you have lost. See that person in your mind in the same manner. Focusing on just the face or the entire person – whichever way you recalled your existing relationship – recall the lost person in the same way. Use the same bright colours. Make the picture just as clear and distinct. Notice the same sounds and voices. Are they moving and breathing? Recall any smells you can relate to that person. Importantly, get back the same physical sensation in your body and recall the sensation of love and happiness that brought. You should now have a strong sense of the person being fully present and with you.

Usually, simply taking the image of the loss experience and moving it to the location of the experience of presence is all that you need to transform the loss. The differences in brightness, colour and movement usually change spontaneously when the location of the image is placed in the same location as the image of the existing relationship. That is simply the way our brains are wired. Simply transform all the sensory memories until the loss experience is fully brought into an experience of presence.

This exercise shows that whether or not you think of someone as absent or present is independent of reality. It is only dependent on how you represent the loved one in your mind, and this is the key to the grief-resolution process.

When this process is complete, you will recover good feelings that you had with the lost person. When this occurs, you may wish to cry, but these tears are very different from the tears of loss. These are tears of reunion, and it is important to allow yourself to take the time to experience these feelings fully.

What If I Don't Want to Get Over My Grief?

Most people are quite happy to transform grief and to reconnect with their lost experiences of love and happiness. Some people, however, do have an issue with resolving grief, and if this is the case, it is an obvious obstacle to recovery. It's worth remembering that grief has value. It is perfectly normal to experience and express grief. In every culture throughout the world there are rituals that encourage and allow us to express grief when we have lost loved ones and it is a natural part of the healing process. These are valuable as they allow us to express deep and powerful feelings.

However, as much as it is important to express grief, it is just as important to let that grief go. Some people believe that if they get over their grief it somehow means letting go of the person and is tantamount to saying goodbye. This is a mistaken notion; this process is not about saying goodbye but rather about saying hello again. You are re-establishing and allowing yourself to again feel the loving connection that you once had with the person.

On the other hand, you may believe that grief is a way to honour someone who has passed on. If you believe this, you might object to letting go of this grief as you would perceive this as dishonouring that person's memory. Of course I agree that you should honour the lost person. But whilst grief is an expression of depth of feeling, it surely honours that person more if you carry them joyfully in your heart with love every day. I'm sure that this person, who loved you, would much prefer you to be happy. It is therefore serving their wishes to recover from grief and bring back your sense of love and happiness.

You may deem perceiving the lost person as being present with you as a form of self-denial, which you might have considered unhelpful. But of course this isn't about denial. Throughout our lives we constantly think about other people, and perhaps even have internal conversations with them. This is about recalling fully and completely the best aspects of the person you loved.

For some reason, you might object to reconnecting with this person as it might interfere with existing relationships that you now have. But I'm sure that you will agree that being preoccupied with grief for this lost person interferes with your existing relationships to a far greater extent. On the other hand, if you can reconnect with this person, you may find that this sense of connection actually supports your existing relationships.

You should be able to proceed with the grief-resolution process, confident that any objection is fully respected, and that your true intention of a positive outcome will be achieved by the process.

Fear

The emotion of fear is associated with the kidneys. The kidneys within Chinese medicine are known as the 'controllers of water'. The human body is approximately 60% water, so the importance of this organ is obviously significant. The kidneys also store 'jing', which is seen in Chinese medicine as our constitutional energy and as controlling our cycles of growth and development, as well as the function of our brains. The kidneys therefore support our mental abilities. The kidneys are also associated with sexual function and sexual problems; infertility is invariably associated with kidney weakness. The kidneys are paired with the bladder, which again has an obvious connection with water.

Chinese medicine associates the following symptoms with an energetic weakness with the kidneys that can be brought about by excessive fear: lower back pain, spinal problems, phobias, lethargy, weak and cold knees, frequent and urgent urination, night sweating, thirst, infertility, poor concentration, poor long-term memory and hearing problems.

It is worth repeating that when we talk about an organ in Chinese medicine we are not merely talking about the organ as Western medicine knows it. Within Chinese medicine many functions and attributes are associated with organs that are not carried out literally by the organ itself. For example, many aspects of the central nervous system and the reproductive system are associated with kidney function.

The conditions that have an association with kidney functioning are Alzheimer's disease, congenital abnormalities, delayed development in children, diabetes, enuresis, hypothyroidism, impotence, infertility, menopause, nephritis, optic neuritis, phobias and tinnitus.

Fear is a normal emotion when we are under threat. If we are threatened, we should do what we can to make ourselves feel safe again. However, when fear lingers, we can be left with an anxiety that leaves us incapacitated. The threat we feel can often be imagined and arise for self-generated perceptions.

A few of us have learned to master fear through experience and time; however, many people live in constant fear for much of their adult lives. In order to overcome fear, you must first learn what it is. The emotion of fear stems from several hormonal and neuro-chemical responses in the brain. The source is there.

We learned earlier on in this chapter about the fight or flight response, when hormones are released throughout the body that begin to trigger defensive mechanisms such as raising adrenaline and cortisol levels, and increasing heart rate and respiration. These symptoms are meant to stay active for only a few seconds or minutes, which is just enough time for a person to react to the object of fear. This protects us and helps us to react quickly in times of danger.

However, what happens when that object or the situation is not real? What if it's simply a situation created by your imagination? In this case, for many people, the high levels of adrenaline and increased cardio-respiratory rates remain in the body for a longer period, creating more stress and consequently making the body experience 'burn-out' and total exhaustion.

The next step in conquering your fear is to actually embrace it. Embracing your fear simply means recognising the symptoms, becoming aware of its presence and devoting your conscious mind to it. Turn your fear into a little experiment. When you start feeling nervous and anxious, put in a conscious effort by taking a moment to say to yourself, 'It's beginning. I'm becoming afraid.' By acknowledging fear and keeping company with it, you will eventually learn how to master it.

The Three Steps to Overcoming Fear

Step One – Embracing Fear

Fear can be a difficult emotion because when you encounter it you are compelled to do something about it. This call to action is part of the reason for fear. But without the ability to be mindful in this situation, this call to action can be premature and even harmful.

The first step is awareness. Your fear is there to protect you. When you feel fear and embrace it mindfully, you can use its energy wisely to find the correct course of action.

Step Two – Acknowledging the Value of Fear

Acknowledging fear is essential if we want to use this emotion wisely. In order to do this, you must become aware about your limiting beliefs about fear and construct a new set of positive beliefs.

Think of fear not as a weakness but as information, a signal of potential risk and a usable energy. Let yourself feel the fear, breathe through it and use its energy. Fear doesn't ever have to become panic. Feel it, let it be and in doing so you can use its energy.

Affirming the value of fear may at first seem wrong, because of the fear-negating culture that we live in. Changing your negative beliefs about fear creates a possibility where fear can exist without damaging your self-esteem or composure.

It's useful to make a list of all the positive aspects of fear. To help you do this, try completing these sentences:

- If fear didn't overwhelm me, I would use its energy to . . .
- Fear equips me with the strength to . . .
- When I see fear as a messenger, I can learn . . .
- I can use fear productively when I . . .

Step Three – Locating Fear in the Body

Fear can produce a profound bodily experience. Now that you have learned to embrace fear, you should have greater composure to notice where in your body you feel fear. Try this experiment.

Sit comfortably and recall a time when you encountered fear. Remember where you were, who was there, what you saw, what you heard, the colours, the smells. Bring the memory back as if it were happening right now. Along with the memory, you should get a sensation in your body. Notice the location of this feeling. Can you describe what colour it is? Usually the sensation is moving – up, down, circling or spiralling.

Having noticed this sensation in all its detail, change the colour and turn the movement of the sensation in a new direction. Breathe deeply and notice how, as you consciously change the direction of the sensation, all feelings of fear dissipate.

In this exercise we recalled a moment of fear. There is no real difference between a recalled moment of fear and an actual moment of fear that can be happening to you in the present. With greater composure, whenever you encounter fear use this exercise to put you back in command.

The NLP Fast Fear Cure

The NLP Fast Fear Cure is a simple yet powerful visualisation developed by Dr Richard Bandler that takes just five or ten minutes. NLP, or neuro-linguistic programming, allows us to hold an owner's manual for our brain. Neuro-linguistic programming describes the fundamental dynamics between mind (neuro) and language (linguistic) and how their interplay affects our body and behaviour (programming). It is designed to cure simple phobias but also to neutralise memories of traumatic experiences such as rape, abuse, combat experiences, etc.

There are two steps to the cure:

Step One

Visualise watching a film of yourself confronting the object of your phobia or going through the experience you have a traumatic memory of.

Two things are critical for this step:

1. You *watch yourself* in the film. For example, if you have a phobia of birds, the film is not just about birds but is about you encountering birds in a way that would be frightening to you. Note that this technique will apply to all phobias you may have.
2. It is crucial that you are able to watch the film and be detached, and in particular to stay out of the film and remain a spectator watching yourself go through the experience. You can check this afterwards by asking yourself, 'So how was it when I watched that film?' If you answer, 'I felt a little afraid,' then ask yourself if you remembered to stay back in your seat in the cinema, or did you actually become involved in the film itself?

   Understandably, it's very difficult for you to remain completely unemotional while imagining watching a film of yourself encountering a situation you are afraid of or have a traumatic memory of. But there are several techniques that are usually very effective in this respect.

   Before the film starts, I want you to float up out of your body into the projection booth, where you can control the film. And as you're in the projection booth, with those enormous reels of film on the projector and that long beam of white light streaming towards the screen, I want you to notice yourself sitting in your seat waiting for the film to start. And now I want you to start the projector and watch yourself as you sit down there in the cinema and watch the film of you going through experience. That's perhaps a bit overly elaborate, but it contains the essential ingredients that usually work. If the subject still can't remain detached, be flexible until you find something that works. Imagine driving on the motorway and seeing the film on the screen of a drive-in in the distance. Have the film shown on a bed sheet that flickers in the wind.

Step Two

When the film is over, imagine stepping into the screen and you are safe. All the birds are gone, or the flight has landed or whatever. Now, with the traumatic part over, see things through your own eyes just as if you were actually there. Things are in colour and three-dimensional. And then very quickly rewind the whole experience to the beginning, like a film rewinding with everything happening in reverse. And then rewind it again even faster. When you can rewind the entire experience in one second repeat, rewind again and again ten times.

Now imagine encountering the fear once more and notice what it feels like. Repeat this exercise until the fear has almost faded into non-existence.

Thought-Field Therapy – Healing Fear

If you are feeling fear or phobias and want to reduce that feeling immediately, you can also use a powerful technique called thought-field therapy, developed by Dr Roger Callahan. Dr Callahan was a practising hypnotherapist, and when he developed this technique, he 'cured' his entire client base within a few short weeks.

Thought-field therapy may seem very strange, but its effectiveness for treating a host of conditions has had extensive scientific verification. By tapping acupuncture points in the exact sequence described, you will move stagnant energy along the meridians, which removes disturbances related to anxieties or addictions. The approach is proven to be effective for overcoming all forms of addiction, craving and anxiety, as well as a host of other conditions. It is important to think about the phobia or fear throughout this exercise.

1. Intentionally concentrate on the fear or phobia that is causing you stress and rate it on a scale of one to ten, with one being a weak fear and ten being strong. Write down the rating so that you can see how much it has reduced at the end of the exercise.
2. Using two fingers of one hand, while still thinking of the fear, tap five times under the eye on the bony part of the cheekbone.

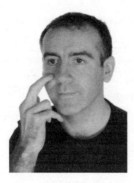

3. Tap solidly five times under the arm, about four inches directly below the armpit.

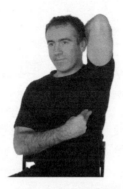

4. Tap the collarbone point five times whilst thinking of the fear. It is found about an inch below the centre of the collarbone.

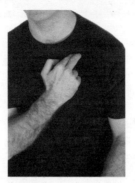

5. Now rate the phobia or fear on a scale of one to ten. If it is still above two, move to the next stage.
6. Now, placing your other hand out in front of you, tap rapidly on the back of your fist between your ring finger and little finger.

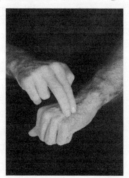

Still thinking of the fear or phobia and whilst continuing to tap rapidly:

- Open and close your eyes.
- Open your eyes and look down to the left.
- Look down to the right.
- Circle your eyes round 360 degrees clockwise.
- Circle your eyes round 360 degrees anticlockwise.
- Hum the first few lines of 'Happy Birthday' out loud.
- Count aloud from one to five.
- Hum a few lines of 'Happy Birthday' again.

7. Tap firmly under the eye again five times.
8. Tap firmly under the arm again five times.
9. Tap firmly under the collarbone again five times.

Now, check how much your fear has decreased. Rate the fear again on the one to ten scale. If the fear hasn't disappeared completely, simply go through the sequence again until it does. Most people will find that they can completely eliminate any fear with just one or two repetitions. Perform the exercise until the fear has disappeared.

Worry

> 'There is nothing that wastes the body like worry, and one who has any faith in God should be ashamed to worry about anything whatsoever.' – Mahatma Gandhi

The emotion of worry is associated with the stomach and spleen in Chinese medicine. These organs essentially represent the digestive system, and their chief function is to assimilate nourishment and energy from the food that we consume. The spleen houses what is called the 'yi', which represents the cognitive mind. Therefore weakness in digestive function commonly manifests in a lack of mental clarity as well as poor energy.

Excessive worry can weaken the digestive function, and the symptoms associated with such spleen and stomach deficiency are poor appetite, stomach discomfort, nausea, diarrhoea, stomach bloating, weak limbs, prolapsed organs, tiredness, obsessive thoughts, muzzy head and poor concentration.

Some illnesses Chinese medicine associates with spleen and stomach deficiency are amnesia, anaemia, anorexia, anxiety, chronic fatigue syndrome, coeliac disease, Crohn's disease, diabetes, food allergies, hernia, hypoglycaemia, hypotension, IBS, leaky gut syndrome, mental fatigue, morning sickness, ME, MS, muscular dystrophy, post-viral syndrome and prolapse.

Worry is really considered 'overthinking'. It is the condition where you are thinking about your feelings instead of feeling your feelings. There is usually a strong proportion of blame present, and this depletes a lot of mental and in turn physical energy.

In fact, our word 'worry' comes from an Old English word meaning 'to strangle' or 'to choke'. Which is what worry does – it can literally choke the life out of us. Medical research has shown that it breaks down our resistance to disease and causes a multitude of health-related problems, particularly in the heart and digestive organs. Short of death and disease, though, worry affects our overall enjoyment of life: it spoils our dispositions, putting us in a perpetual bad mood; it hurts our relationships by making us bad company to be around; and it robs us of zest, energy and optimism.

It's irresponsible to worry because it wastes our energy and leaves us without the resources we need for truly constructive and creative problem-solving. Worry wears us out and drags us down, so that we don't have what it takes to deal with the issues that really should concern us. As one reformed worrier put it, 'Worry doesn't empty the day of its trouble, but only of its strength.'

Worry is irrelevant because it doesn't do you any good. It can't change anything. It can't remedy anything. It can't help anything. Think about it this way:

- An estimated 40% of things we worry about will never actually happen.
- A further 30% are things from the past that can't possibly be changed.
- About 12% are to do with our health (when nothing is actually wrong with us).
- And 10% are too petty and insignificant to matter.
- That means that only 8% of the things we worry about legitimately deserve our thought and concern, but even still, expending energy worrying usually does little or nothing to rectify the situation.

Worry is irrelevant, it's irresponsible, it's pointless, and it potentially does an enormous amount of harm. So what can we do to overcome worry?

The Worry-dissolving Exercise

This exercise removes habitual worry and promotes a more positive and optimistic mental state.

Step One

Think of the thing that is worrying you. The nature of a worry is that we contemplate a future event as if it has already happened. We imagine an accident that could happen, an exam we might fail, not being able to cope with something, etc.

Step Two

When you think about your worry, notice what image you create in your head, any thoughts and any feelings you create. You might imagine seeing an accident in full colour in front of you and hear the screech of car tyres and feel your stomach churning.

Step Three

Now ask yourself if this worry helps you. If the answer is yes, then define how exactly it is useful. For example, in the case of the accident you might take precautions to avoid it happening. You might wear your seat belt. Once you have written down and acknowledged all the benefits of the worry, there is no longer any point in worrying.

Step Four

Now imagine the image of worry being placed on a screen. You can now see the worry and hear the sounds as if it is happening on a film. Imagine placing this screen up and to your left.

Step Five

Now imagine the future as if the worry has actually manifested. See yourself on another screen coping very well with the outcome. When observing this image, notice that you have also taken action as a result of Step Three in order to protect yourself. As a result see yourself smiling and looking calm and relaxed. Place this screen up and to your right.

Step Six

Now, with your mind, imagine taking the screen with the original worry from the left and placing it right in front of you. Counting down – three, two, one – imagine the screen fading into the distance as the second screen (with the positive image) sweeps in and replaces the negative image. It is important to do this rapidly. Repeat this step five times or until the original worry is significantly diminished.

In Summary

- Emotional health is a key component of physical and mental well-being. When recovering health, we often overlook this important component of the Healing Code.
- Mental health and emotional health are not the same thing. An individual may well have the ability to deal with high levels of stress and function in a very effective manner. However, he may present a façade of being in complete control of his life. He may have strong mental resilience to deal with the most difficult of issues. This same person, however, could be suffering from an emotional disorder.
- An emotional disorder can be seen as any reaction or action that does not allow an individual to admit his or her true feelings regarding a situation. Based on this definition, depression is a mental and physical disorder but not an emotional disorder. An emotional disorder, such as repressed emotions of anger and frustration, can however precipitate the onset of the depressed state. This is acknowledged by Western and Eastern psychologists alike.
- We also know people who seem to be devoid of all emotion. Whilst this might appear like a good thing, it is often symptomatic of emotional repression, which in fact is quite detrimental to the individual's health. Suppression of emotion can

ultimately lead to both mental and physical consequences. When a person refuses to acknowledge emotional feelings, this can grow and develop into something more problematic.

- The exercises in this chapter cannot erase events that have happened in your past that may have caused you emotional distress. That is simply impossible. They can, however, alter your perception of these events. Our lives are not a consequence of our previous experiences. More to the point, we are who we are because of the perception of these experiences. In addition to helping you alter your perception, the exercises in this chapter can give you the opportunity to express and release emotions that were experienced in the past.

- By allowing yourself to experience emotion, emotional health can be restored. By reflecting inwards, you can determine what emotional issues have been stored in the memory of your body's cells. Once you understand how denial of emotion can cause illnesses to manifest, this approach will often become an important component of preventative medicine and indeed health recovery.

The Healing Code has now addressed the thoughts and emotions that you encounter each and every day. These emotions have affected your health. Freeing your capacity for powerful, positive thoughts and emotions supports your health recovery. You are now more in control of your emotions, rather than your emotions being in control of you. It is time now to turn our attention to a fundamental third step of your health recovery – the food that you eat.

CHAPTER FOUR

Step Three: The Healing Code Nutrition Plan

The Role of Nutrition

When I was first diagnosed with MS I considered many aspects of my life, one of which included the food I ate. If someone asked me at that time if I had a good diet, I would have said yes, because I did eat what I considered to be a lot of nutritious food. However, I also ate a lot of poor-quality 'junk' food. As I said earlier, people I worked with called me the human dustbin and I had somehow deluded myself that this was OK, as if the good foods were somehow compensating for the junk. In my practice, I have noticed that most people think that they are eating a relatively healthy balanced diet, but upon closer examination, this is rarely the case. I have to assume that people are either so confused that they don't know what a healthy eating plan is or else they are just self-deluding.

It was logical to me that the food I was putting into my body every day had a huge influence on my health. I carried out extensive research to find out which foods were optimum for my condition and completely revamped my eating habits. Within just eight short weeks I felt completely different both in mind and body and had a greater sense of vitality than I had enjoyed for many years. This vitality has continued to grow as I have maintained the eating plan.

When I then began researching what nutrition elements were optimum for other health conditions, it soon became obvious that there was a great deal of similarity between the foods optimum for fighting heart disease, overcoming and preventing cancer, combating diabetes and battling MS, as well as a whole host of other conditions. This brings us to the third step of the Healing Code – nutrition. The Healing Code Nutrition Plan draws together the common aspects of all these food strategies and prepares your body for optimum self-healing.

Hippocrates, the 'Father of Medicine', said, 'Let your food be your medicine and your medicine be your food.' The Healing Code Nutrition Plan is at the core of our overall programme for rapid health recovery. It's simply a fact that nutrition plays a direct role in the development of most illnesses and is therefore a direct cause of most deaths. Doesn't it seem strange therefore that a thorough understanding of nutrition is not a fundamental requisite of all medical practitioners? Most doctors have had little exposure to nutrition training in medical school, and it is only recently that medical students have been exposed to the vital role that nutrition plays in our health. Let's remember that apart from the air we breathe, the only other source of healthy input into our bodies comes from what we eat and drink. It is therefore absolutely logical that the food that you eat and the food you avoid are going to play a direct role in surging your body rapidly back to full health. When it comes to nutrition, there are no half measures and so we will follow the plan to the full. This will ensure that your full recovery is optimised by the foods you are eating.

The Healing Code Nutrition Plan regenerates your body and empowers your health by surging your body with nutrients. The plan combines the optimum food strategies for treating all major health conditions. To prevent or correct most degenerative diseases, the Healing Code Nutrition Plan therefore offers the ideal way to eat.

Demystifying the Alchemy of Nutrition

There are a number of books on the market that advocate varied strategies for weight loss. Many of these gain much media attention, particularly when they promote a controversial approach to nutrition. Unfortunately, many of these approaches are based on little or no scientific evidence. However, it might surprise you to learn that there has been recent broad medical consensus as to what foods are preferred for recovering health. This growing convergence of opinion from the world's leading nutritional scientists has led to the Healing Code Nutrition Plan, developed from information supplied by the world's leading nutritional scientists and backed by much evidence-based research.

The foods selected as part of the plan have been proven by clinical studies to combat a wide variety of diseases. As part of the plan we will encourage the increased intake of antioxidant foods, which play a direct role in the protection against illness and premature ageing.

Free Radicals and the Role of Antioxidants

Denham Harman, MD, developed the free-radical theory of ageing at the University of Nebraska in 1956. Free radicals are abnormal molecules with a missing electron that hence create a negative charge. They are unstable and highly reactive because they are always seeking to find the missing electron in their structure by bonding with nearby 'normal' molecules.

Many things accelerate the production of free radicals, including chemical toxins, diet, alcohol, smoking, radiation and excessive exercise. Creating free radicals is unavoidable, and the simple acts of living, breathing, eating and drinking all play a part in their production. Free radicals are simply a natural by-product of cell metabolism. However, though natural, they are harmful to your body's cells and they can accelerate ageing if they are present in large amounts. Harman recognised that free radicals are the main culprits that destroy cell structure.

So how can we protect ourselves against free radicals? Enter antioxidants. Antioxidant nutrients help your body to neutralise free radicals and hence fight against ageing and ill health. They are stable molecules that neutralise the free radicals by donating one of their own electrons to them.

Luckily, thanks to their original structure, by giving away one electron, the antioxidants themselves don't become unstable. Think of them as scavengers that help prevent cell and tissue damage that could lead to age-related diseases. In order to protect against the damage of free radicals, it is necessary to take a wide variety of antioxidants. Important antioxidants include beta carotene, coenzyme Q10, grapeseed extract and vitamins C and E. A fundamental aspect of the Healing Code Nutrition Plan is that it is very high in these important antioxidants and therefore helps in the fight against illness.

The Healing Code Nutrition Plan Key Principles

The eight points that make up the principles of the Healing Code Nutrition Plan are broadly accepted by leading medical authorities both within Western and Eastern medicine. The following are the main principles of the plan:

- Replace bad fats – saturated and trans fats – with good fats. Eliminate all processed foods containing trans fatty acids.
- Eliminate dairy products containing 1% butterfat or more and replace with soya or rice milk.
- Eliminate refined carbohydrates including sugar, white bread and pasta.
- Replace red and dark meat with healthier sources of protein.
- Consume large quantities of organic fruit and vegetables.
- Drink plenty of water and restrict alcohol consumption to a maximum of one glass of red wine per day.
- Replace coffee and tea with green and jasmine tea.
- Replace refined table salt with healthy spices.

Although the the Healing Code Nutrition Plan is based on modern scientific evidence, it is remarkably similar to the diet of our ancient ancestors, which contained all of these elements. Below is a quick breakdown of the essentials:

Replace	With
Red and brown meat	Chicken, fish and vegetable protein
Butter	Organic extra-virgin olive oil
Milk (full fat and semi-skimmed)	Skimmed milk or organic soya milk
Chocolate	Raisins and dried fruit
Sugar	Moderate amounts of organic honey
Soft drinks	Fresh juices and water
Beer	Red wine (max. one glass per day)
Coffee and tea	Green tea or jasmine tea
White bread	Wholemeal bread
Table salt	Spices

Changing Your Eating Habits

Let's face it, changing your eating habits, like any changes in life, causes some discomfort. Whilst recognising this, converting from eating poor-quality foods to optimum nutrition for health recovery is perhaps one of the most powerful things you can do to fight your way back to health. When you fight back, you obviously want to do so with the maximum impact and therefore if a radical change in eating habits is required, then let it be so. The good news is that if a radical change is required, the gains to you are likely to be even more dramatic.

When I radically changed my diet, I gave up many foods that until that time I thought were part of who I was. I therefore needed to develop a system and utilise techniques to alter my behaviour to eating. These powerful techniques can be applied to all aspects that are toxic to the self-healing process – whether it is harmful food cravings, nicotine addiction, alcohol addiction or even utilisation of things in your lifestyle that are harmful to your health. These

121

extraordinary techniques will make up the fourth step on our journey – the Healing Code Detox. We will therefore look at ways to put the eating plan into practice in Chapter Five, but for now let's focus on the principles of the Healing Code Nutrition Plan.

The following table gives a comprehensive listing of many of the most popular foods, along with suggestions as to how freely you should eat each food. Where there is a tick, this means the food is a good choice; you are free to eat this food in any permissible amount. Where there is a cross, you should avoid this food completely, as it is likely to slow your health recovery.

✓　= good choice
✗　= avoid completely
◆　= caution – limited intake
A　= anti-cancer
B　= high in antioxidants
C　= antiviral
D　= high in refined carbohydrates

◆	Alfalfa	A	Thought to protect against breast cancer, reduces inflammation, however avoid with auto-immune diseases
✓	Apple	A	Lowers cholesterol and relieves constipation
✓	Apricots	A	Used frequently by Chinese medicine to treat cancer, improves circulation, natural laxative
✓	Artichokes	B	Supports liver function and improves digestion
✓	Asparagus	B	Stimulates the kidneys
✓	Aubergine	B, C	Helps prevent strokes and haemorrhages. Protects against cholesterol damage
✓	Avocado	B	Good blood tonic
✗	Bagel	D	Eat only wholewheat bagels
✗	Baked Beans	D	High in sugar
◆	Banana	C	Limit intake – high in potassium and has antibiotic qualities, but can be problematic for diabetics. Can cause acid residues

✓	Barley	A, B	Reduces cholesterol. Supports liver and digestive function
✓	Bean Curd (Tofu)	A, B C	Helps to lower cholesterol
✗	Beef		High in saturated fat
✓	Beetroot	A, B	A rich source of vitamins and minerals. Supports detoxification and strengthens blood
✗	Biscuits	D	High in trans fats
✓	Black Beans	A, B	Lowers cholesterol. Good source of fibre and protein
✓	Bok choi	A, B	Stimulates immunity and improves digestion
✓	Broccoli	A, B, C	Supports liver function and intestinal cleanser
✓	Brown Rice		A healthier alternative to white rice, high in vitamins and minerals. Calms nervous system and lifts mood
✓	Brussels Sprouts	A, B	Supports pancreatic function. Protects against a variety of cancers
✓	Buckwheat		High in fibre and protein
✓	Butter Beans	A, B	Lowers cholesterol. Good source of fibre and protein
✓	Cabbage	A, B	Stimulates immunity and improves digestion
✗	Cakes	D	High in trans fats
✓	Carrots	A, B	High in beta carotene
✓	Cashew Nuts	B	Only choose unsalted cashew nuts. Lowers cholesterol
✓	Cauliflower	A, B	Supports kidney and bladder function
✓	Celery	A, B	Supports digestion and lowers blood pressure
✗	Cereal Bars	D	High in sugar and trans fats
✗	Cheese		High in saturated fat
✓	Cherries (fresh)	B	Strengthens immunity and relieves headaches
✓	Chicken		Choose only organic free-range chicken and eat only lean chicken breast
✗	Chicken Nuggets		High in trans fats and saturated fats
✓	Chickpeas	B	Anti-inflammatory and supports digestive and kidney function. Excellent source of protein
◆	Chillies		Limit intake – can cause inflammation of the stomach
✓	Chives	A, B, C	Lowers cholesterol
✗	Chocolate	D	High in saturated fats

✗	Coffee		High in caffeine which can cause a variety of health problems. Decaf coffee should also be avoided because of potentially harmful chemicals
✗	Cola drinks	D	Exceptionally high in sugar
✗	Commercial Breakfast Cereals	D	Generally avoid as most contain excessive sodium, sugar and other refined carbohydrates
✓	Corn	A, B	High in good fats and supports nervous system function
✗	Corn Flakes	D	High in sugar
✓	Courgette	B	Contains vitamins A, B and C and can alleviate bladder and kidney infections
✓	Cranberries	B, C	Supports bladder and kidney function
✗	Croissant	D	High in trans fats
✓	Cucumber	B	Supports digestion as well as kidney and bladder function
✗	Custard	D	High in sugar
✓	Dates	A	Used to treat respiratory conditions
✗	Diet Soft Drinks		Avoid completely – contains artificial sweeteners which may damage the central nervous system
✗	Digestive Biscuits	D	High in trans fats and sugar
✗	Duck		High in saturated fat
◆	Eggs		Limit to 4 eggs per week. Good source of protein, iron, selenium, vitamins B and D, but raises cholesterol. Only choose organic free-range eggs
✓	Fennel	A	Helps prevent blood clotting and supports digestive function
✓	Fish (oily)		High in omega 3 EFA and protects against a wide variety of conditions
✗	French Fries		High in trans and saturated fats
◆	Fruit Juice		Avoid commercial fruit juices; make your own juices from organic fruit
✓	Garlic	A, C	Lowers cholesterol, decongestant and prevents blood clotting
✓	Grapefruit	A, B	Lowers cholesterol, supports cardio vascular function. Fights allergies and throat and mouth infections

✓	Grapes	B	Good blood tonic
✓	Green Beans	B	Boosts white blood cell count immunity
✗	Ham		High in saturated fat
✗	Hamburger		High in saturated fat and trans fats
◆	Honey		Moderate intake of organic honey is a good replacement for sugar
✓	Houmous	A	High in protein and fibre
✗	Ice Cream	D	Contains dairy and high in sugar
✗	Jam	D	Exceptionally high in sugar
✗	Jelly	D	High in sugar
✓	Kale	A, B	Helps regulate hormones
✓	Kidney Beans	A, B	Supports digestive function
✓	Kiwi	A, B	Used in Chinese medicine to treat cancer. Supports digestive function
✗	Lamb		High in saturated fat
✓	Leeks	B	Supports detoxification
✓	Lemon	A, B	Strengthens immune function
✓	Lentils	A	High in folic acid
✓	Lettuce		Rich in fibre and vitamins. Suports bones and joints
✓	Lime	A, B	Strengthens immune function
◆	Liquorice	A	Limit intake of real liquorice, has anti-cancer properties and kills bacteria. Avoid if experiencing raised blood pressure or pregnant. Supports digestive function. These benefits do not apply to liquorice sweets
✓	Mango	A, B, C	Antibacterial and immuno-boosting. Supports kidney and digestive function
✗	Marmalade	D	Exceptionally high in sugar
✗	Milk, Full Fat		High in saturated fat and weakens digestion
✗	Milk, Semi-skimmed		High in saturated fat and weakens digestion
✓	Milk, Skimmed		Permissible. Also consider organic soya milk
✗	Muffins	D	High in trans fats, saturated fats and sugar
✓	Mung Beans	A, B	Good blood cleanser and supports detoxification
✓	Mushrooms	A	Shiitake mushrooms are used to treat a wide variety of conditions. Supports immunity
◆	Noodles		Choose only organic whole wheat noodles

✓	Oats	B	Good choice – high in antioxidants and lowers cholesterol. Some people are intolerant to oats however and if you experience bloating or digestive problems you are best to avoid
✓	Onions	A, B, C	Natural antibiotic. Supports detoxification
✓	Orange	A, B	High in vitamin C and supports digestion
✓	Orange Juice		Good choice when juiced at home. Avoid processed juices
✓	Parsnips	A, B	Supports kidney and digestive function
✓	Pasta		Choose only organic whole wheat pasta
✓	Peach (fresh)	B	Supports detoxification, rich in minerals
✓	Peanuts (unsalted)		High in good fats, vitamins and minerals. Eat only unsalted peanuts
✓	Pear	B	High in iodine and benefits thyroid function. Supports digestion and detoxification
✓	Peas		Good source of vegetable protein. Source of calcium. Supports liver function
✓	Peppers	B	Good choice – high in antioxidants and vitamin C
✓	Pineapple	C	Suppresses inflammation. Antibacterial qualities
✓	Pinto Beans	A, B	High in protein and dietary fibre
◆	Pitta Bread		Eat only wholemeal pitta bread
✗	Pizza	D	Avoid completely – high in saturated fat
✓	Plum	C	Good source of fibre. Supports blood circulation and digestion
✗	Popcorn	D	High in salt and refined carbohydrates
✗	Pork		High in saturated fat
✓	Porridge	B	Lowers cholesterol. Some people are intolerant to oats however and if you experience bloating or digestive problems you are best to avoid
◆	Potatoes	A	Limit intake – anticancer properties but as it raises insulin levels you should eat in moderation particularly if trying to lose weight
✗	Pretzels	D	Avoid completely – high in salt and refined carbohydrates

✓	Prunes		High in fibre. Supports blood and central nervous system. Helps to lower cholesterol
✓	Pumpkin	A, B	High in beta carotene, protects against heart disease
✓	Radishes	B	Expectorant which reduces mucus and helps to clear sinuses. Supports digestion
✓	Raisins	B	High in vitamins and minerals
◆	Rhubarb	B	High in vitamins B, C, iron and calcium. Lowers cholesterol. Acidic, so avoid if dealing with kidney stones, gout, gallstones or cancer
✓	Rice	A, B	Choose only brown rice – high in vitamins, minerals and fibre. Lowers cholesterol and inhibits the development of kidney stones
✓	Rocket	A, B	Stimulates appetite and supports digestion
✓	Rye Bread		High in dietary fibre and complex carbohydrates. Benefits the liver and supports digestion
✗	Salami	B	Avoid completely – high in saturated fat
◆	Salmon	B	Only eat wild salmon as farmed salmon has been shown to contain cancer-causing polychlorinated biphenyls, or PCBs, that exceed health guidelines. Rich in omega-3 essential fatty acids. Boosts immunity
✓	Sardines	B	Good choice – high in omega-3 EFAs and protects against a wide variety of conditions
✗	Sausages		Avoid completely – high in saturated fat
✗	Scallops		Avoid completely – prone to toxic contamination
✓	Sesame Seeds	B	Lowers cholesterol. Rich in omega-3 and -6 EFAs. Benefits cardiovascular and nervous systems
✓	Shallots	A, B	Protects against blood clotting
✗	Shellfish (prawn, crab, lobster)		Avoid completely – prone to toxic contamination
✗	Soft Drinks		Avoid completely – contains extremely high amounts of refined sugar
✓	Soy Beans	A, B, C	Helps to lower cholesterol
✓	Soya Milk	A, B, C	Good choice – anticancer properties – only use organic soya milk

✓	Spaghetti		Choose only organic whole wheat spaghetti
✓	Spinach	A, B	High in beta carotene. Regulates blood pressure and supports immunity and bone health
✓	Spring Onions	A, B, C	Help prevent tumour and cancer formations Supports digestion and blood circulation Strengthens bones and joints
✗	Steak		High in saturated fat
✓	Strawberries	A, B, C	Good choice – antiviral and anticancer properties
✗	Stuffing, Bread	D	High in saturated fats and trans fats
✗	Sugar	D	Avoid completely – causes a variety of health problems
✓	Sultanas	B	High in vitamins and minerals
✓	Sweet Potato	B	High in beta carotene
◆	Tea, English		Limit intake – high caffeine content
✓	Tea, Green	A, B	Excellent choice – high in antioxidants and has anticancer properties
✓	Tea, Jasmine	A, B	Excellent choice – high in antioxidants and has anticancer properties
✓	Tofu	A, B, C	Helps to lower cholesterol
✓	Tomato	A, B	Antiseptic. Reduces liver inflammation
✓	Trout	B	Good choice – high in omega-3 EFA and protects against a wide variety of conditions
✓	Tuna	B	Good choice – high in omega-3 EFA and protects against a wide variety of conditions
✓	Turkey		Good choice – low in saturated fat. Only eat the white meat of turkey
✗	Veal		Avoid completely – high in saturated fat
◆	Vinegar		Limit intake particularly if suffering from digestive disorders. Use lemon juice as an alternative
✗	Waffles	D	Avoid completely – high in trans fats
✓	Watercress	A, B	Good choice – antioxidant and anticancer properties. Stimulates the appetite and acts as a tonic
✓	Watermelon	A, B	Good source of potassium
◆	Wheat	A	High incidence of intolerance towards wheat so avoid if you experience bloating or digestive problems. If not wheat does have good anticancer properties

✗　White Bread　　　D　　High in trans fats and refined carbohydrates

✓　Wholemeal Bread　　　　Good choice – but avoid if you show signs of
intolerance – bloating indigestion etc.

◆　Yoghurt　　　　　A　　Limit – only choose live organic low saturated
fat varieties. Antibacterial and anticancer
properties. Contains acidophilus bacteria

The Healing Code Nutrition Plan Key Principles Explained

Good Fats and Bad Fats

> Replace bad fats – saturated and trans fats – with good fats.
> Eliminate all processed foods containing trans fatty acids.

You may be aware that there are many different forms of fat, some of which are considered good for you and others that are considered bad, but do you know which ones are which? It's important to know the answer to this because, putting it simply, bad fats can cause serious damage to your health, whilst good fats will help to return your body back to full health.

Two fats are generally considered 'bad'. These are trans fats and saturated fats. There is such strong evidence against both fats – particularly trans fats – that the Healing Code Nutrition Plan sensibly encourages the reduction of saturated-fat intake and the elimination of trans-fat intake.

Trans Fats

Trans fats are found in many processed foods, including biscuits, solid and semi-solid margarines, commercial cooking oils and many domestic cooking oils. Look closely at any processed-food labels that you buy. If you see 'hydrogenated' or 'partially hydrogenated' on the label, simply put it right back on the shelf.

129

Hydrogenated fats are produced by taking liquid oil and putting it through a process called hydrogenation. This process combines heat and pressure to add several hydrogen atoms to the oil. It takes place over several hours in the presence of a nickel or platinum catalyst and converts the liquid to a semi solid.

Hydrogenation helps prevent the oil from becoming rancid but destroys its nutritional value. This process enables manufacturers to convert cheap low-quality oils into butter substitutes, hence the explosion of margarines on the market. It has nothing to do with improving health and everything to do with producing low-class, low-cost food for profit. The fact that this stuff is detrimental to your health is neither here nor there to the food manufacturer that produces this junk.

Hydrogenation also produces a residue of toxic metals, including aluminium and nickel. These metals accumulate in our cells and nervous system, where they poison enzyme systems and alter cellular functions, endangering health and causing a wide variety of problems.

Because trans fats don't occur naturally, our bodies are simply not designed to deal with them effectively and they hence become poisonous to crucial cellular reactions. The trans-fat measurement in human red blood cells has been shown to be as high as 20%. This figure should in fact be zero. While red blood cells were used in this measurement because they're easy to access, it is safe to assume that most other cell membranes in the body also contain these toxic fats.

So what is the end result of consuming these trans fats? The cell membranes weaken, which in turn alters the normal transport of minerals and other nutrients across the membrane. This results in disease and toxic chemicals invading the cells more easily. The result is sick, weak cells, poor organ function and damaged immune function – in short, dramatically increased risk of disease.

Another problem with trans fats is that they inhibit our body's ability to eliminate cholesterol. Normally our liver puts any excess cholesterol into bile and then transfers it to the gall bladder, before moving it to the small intestine. Trans fats block this normal conversion of cholesterol in the liver, which results in elevated cholesterol levels in the blood. This causes an increase in the amount of low-density lipoproteins (LDLs, or bad cholesterol), considered to be one of the chief contributors to arterial disease. The double whammy is that trans fats also lower high-density lipoproteins (HDLs, or good cholesterol), which normally act to protect the heart and cardiovascular system from the negative effects of the LDLs.

Trans fats also increase production of the body's pro-inflammatory hormones and inhibit production of the anti-inflammatory hormones. As a result, we are more vulnerable to inflammatory conditions and we can develop problems with allergic reactions, blood pressure, clotting, cholesterol levels, hormone activity and immune function.

There is a burgeoning amount of scientific evidence indicating that trans fats contribute to heart disease, cancer, diabetes, immunity and reproduction problems, as well as obesity. A Harvard Medical School study followed more than eighty-five thousand women over an eight-year period. The researchers compared the diets of those who developed heart disease over that time with those who did not. They found that major dietary sources of trans fats, such as margarine, were significantly associated with higher risks of coronary heart disease.

Because of the known health effects of by-products of hydrogenation, there is no doubt that government health regulations would not allow the process to be used for making edible products if it were to be introduced today.

So be sure to read the labels on packaged foods, and always make sure to avoid those with hydrogenated or partially hydrogenated oil. Because most food labels do not include the amount of trans fats on the nutritional information, it is wise to look for 'partially hydrogenated' vegetable oils. If this is listed as one of the first three ingredients, it usually indicates the product contains substantial amounts of trans fats.

Saturated Fats

Saturated fats are found in some of the most common foods: butter, cream, cheese, chocolate, coconut and red meat.

We know that when saturated fats are cut to extremely low levels, cholesterol levels can drop precipitously. This dietary change can achieve dramatic results, and people should minimise their intake of saturated fats, which play a role in raising bad cholesterol (LDLs) and increasing the risk of cardiovascular disease.

Saturated fats are non-essential fats. This means that our body does not need them added to our diet. Animal fats and chocolate found in dairy and meat are high in a saturated fat called stearic acid. Although scientists have found that whilst stearic may not raise LDL levels, it still increases inflammation, an emerging risk factor in cardiovascular-disease development, as well as in cancer and many other diseases.

Saturated fats, which are solid at room temperature, have other negative effects. These fats can replace the more positive unsaturated fats in the body's cells, which are liquid at room temperature and become incorporated into cell membranes. This makes these more rigid, causing malfunctions leading to, among other things, insulin resistance.

Several large scientific studies have confirmed that when we replace saturated fat with unsaturated oils, we can achieve up to a 65% reduction in heart-disease deaths.

Treatment with statin drugs, which lower LDL cholesterol, seem only to be half as effective as this dietary change because these drugs don't address all the risks.

Good Fats

Fat is also, however, an important part of a healthy diet. There is strong evidence that many 'good' fats actually reduce the risk of heart attack and stroke. Good fats help sugar and insulin metabolism and therefore contribute to our goals of long-term weight loss and weight maintenance.

Good fats include monounsaturated fats, found in extra-virgin olive oil and canola oil, nuts and avocados. Monounsaturated fats actually lower total and LDL cholesterol – which accumulates in and clogs artery walls – while maintaining levels of HDL cholesterol, which carries cholesterol from the artery walls and delivers it to the liver for disposal.

Monounsaturated fats are essential for our cells to function normally. The fatty acids are involved in countless chemical processes in our bodies and are used as building blocks for certain hormones.

Two types of fatty acids – omega-3 and omega-6 – cannot be made by our bodies and therefore must be obtained through the foods or supplements we have in our diets. They are called essential fatty acids (EFAs), and there is evidence that they have been helpful to many people with allergies, anaemia, arthritis, cancer, candida, depression, diabetes, eczema, fatigue, heart disease, inflammation, multiple sclerosis, premenstrual syndrome (PMS), psoriasis, sluggish metabolism and viral infections.

Omega-3 fatty acids – polyunsaturated fats found in coldwater fish, canola oil, flaxseed, walnuts and almonds – also count as good fat. Studies have proven that people who eat more omega-3s have fewer serious health problems such as heart disease and diabetes. There is also strong evidence that omega-3 oils help prevent or treat depression, arthritis and asthma, as well as a host of other conditions.

Studies have also shown that healthy women who ate fish at least five times a week had a 45% lower risk of developing life-threatening heart disease. Another study showed that men who had experienced a heart attack when randomly assigned fish-oil supplements (1 g a day) had a 53% decrease in mortality.

Omega-6 oils are primarily found in vegetables and seeds. A deficiency of omega-6 essential fatty acids can result in auto-immune problems, breast pain, eczema, hypertension and inflammation.

The message is clear: eating more seafood is of considerable benefit to your health. The Healing Code Nutrition Plan therefore recommends at least three servings of oily fish per week, together with adequate portions of leafy green vegetables. If you dislike fish, there are other options, such as flaxseed, canola and soy oils as well as flaxseeds, walnuts and soybeans. If you do not eat fish, I suggest you take a good-quality fish-oil supplement (1 g) per day.

Always remember to refrigerate your oils after opening. Also, if they are not in lightproof bottles, keep them out of the direct light.

Dairy Products

Eliminate dairy products and replace with soya or rice milk.

Going dairy-free will change how you look and how you feel, as well as adding years to your life. A lot of people might be taken aback by this statement. That's not surprising, as the dairy industry has been successful in convincing many of us that dairy products are necessary for sustaining good health. This claim does not stand up to any close scrutiny, and the reality is that full-fat dairy products are clearly detrimental to our health.

Cow's milk is meant for calves, and babies are meant to drink their mother's milk until weaned from it. Nature has designed both types of milk and digestive systems accordingly. Humans are the only mammals that drink milk once they have reached adulthood, and even more stupidly, we drink the milk of a completely different species that is ten times our size. We consume vast amounts of this dairy slime and fool ourselves that it is good for us.

Let's look at the facts again. A calf has four stomachs and nine feet of intestines. We have 27 feet of intestines. Our digestive system is not designed to break down a food that is meant to nurse the young of another species. Our stomachs therefore find it extremely difficult to digest dairy food.

Remember that cows are injected with large amounts of steroids and antibiotics, which automatically get passed on to their milk. Most cows also graze on pesticide-infested grass. The milk therefore can become loaded with pus from cows that have mastitis, which is also treated with antibiotics. Despite the numerous drugs the cows are treated with, not all the bacteria can be destroyed.

Moreover, butterfat – the fat in whole milk that becomes highly concentrated in cream, ice cream, cheese and, of course, butter – is the most saturated of the animal fats, delivering a massive 54% of saturated fatty acids. Butterfat in the Western diet, particularly in the form of cheese, is probably the greatest single contributor to the overload of saturated fat responsible for the high rates of cardiovascular disease in our societies.

Cow's milk has four times the protein and only half the carbohydrate content of human milk; pasteurisation destroys the natural enzyme in cow's milk required to digest its heavy protein content. This excess milk protein therefore putrefies in the human digestive tract, clogging the intestines with sticky sludge, some of which seeps into the bloodstream. As this putrid sludge accumulates from daily consumption of dairy products, the body forces some of it out through the skin (causing acne and blemishes) and lungs (causing catarrh), while the rest of it festers inside, forms mucus and breeds infections, causes allergic reactions and stiffens joints with calcium deposits. Many cases of chronic asthma, allergies, ear infections and acne have been totally cured simply by eliminating all dairy products from the diet.

From a traditional Chinese medical perspective, dairy products are considered the most 'damp' foods. Eating 'damp' foods, especially in the context of a 'damp' climate tends to give rise to 'damp' illnesses. Examples of damp illnesses are bronchitis, asthma, multiple sclerosis, coronary heart disease and cancer. It is notable that the incidences of these illnesses are much higher in countries where consumption of full-fat dairy products is high.

Shortly after my MS diagnosis I gave up all dairy products by following the Swank Diet. I mentioned earlier that when I was growing up I remember laughing at the suggestion that you should breathe in through your nose and out through your mouth. This to me was silly because I thought it was simply impossible to breathe through your nose. Within four weeks of giving up dairy products I could breathe air through my nostrils, for the first time since I could remember. Dairy products are 'damp', or mucus-forming. This mucus builds up and starts to compromise your breathing by filling your sinuses. As mucus is also found in our digestive system, eating dairy products will have a significantly detrimental effect on digestion. If you react in any negative way to food that you eat, you don't have to be Sherlock Holmes to figure out what your body is telling you to do.

Many people falsely believe that they have to eat dairy products for calcium and to prevent osteoporosis. The US is one of the largest consumers of dairy products, but isn't it strange that 25 million American women over the age of 40 have been diagnosed with arthritis and osteoporosis? Studies have shown that on average these women consumed 2 lb of milk per day for their entire adult lives. The truth is that osteoporosis rates are much lower in societies where people do not eat dairy products. For every gramme of protein that you eat you will lose up to 2 mg of calcium in your urine. The high protein content of dairy products tends to leach calcium from our bodies. Although cow's milk contains calcium, it also contains large amounts of phosphorus. Phosphorus combines with calcium in the digestive tract and actually blocks its assimilation. Consequently cow's milk is not as good a source of calcium as other more digestible foods, such as broccoli, kale, sesame seeds, dates, figs, prunes, kelp and sardines. Remember that cows get their calcium simply from eating grass.

If you find you are really struggling to completely eliminate all dairy products from your diet, it is acceptable to consume a small amount of skimmed (not semi-skimmed or full-fat) milk, but do try to replace this with organic soya milk over time. If you can find it, you can also eat cheese that contains less than 1% butterfat, although I have found it hard to source this outside of the US. I recommend replacing cheese with hummus or tofu.

Refined Carbohydrates — the Man-made Poison

Eliminate refined carbohydrates including sugar, white bread and pasta.

Refined carbohydrates are the high-insulin-producing, fat-causing, energy-destroying, stomach-bloating foods that have been artificially created by man. Refined carbs include baked goods (muffins, doughnuts, pastries, biscuits, cakes), white flour and white-flour products (white bread and bagels), snack foods (sweets, crisps, pretzels), sweetened dairy products (ice cream, chocolate milk), drinks (pop/soda, concentrated fruit juice), processed grain products (pasta made from white flour, white rice, rice cakes, many breakfast cereals).

Refined carbohydrates are generally considered bad news. They have little nutritional value and are in fact detrimental to our health. They are commonly found in most processed foods. These carbohydrates wreak havoc with your digestion and turn your blood sugar into a roller coaster of highs and lows, which in turn can cause a host of nasty things to happen throughout your body. One particular nasty culprit is high-fructose corn syrup, which is found in a wide variety of foods, including ketchup, juices and breakfast cereals. The Healing Code Nutrition Plan recommends that you avoid all processed foods for this amongst other reasons.

White flour is also a refined carbohydrate, so you should try to avoid white bread, cakes and biscuits made from flour.

The Healing Code Nutrition Plan substitutes whole grains and fruit and vegetables for refined carbohydrates. These whole grains are higher in beneficial fibre, vitamins and, in the case of fruit and vegetables, other useful phytonutrients. This means that they are not only more nutritious in general, but they also help to control and sustain normal energy levels and appetite more effectively. A diet high in whole grains decreases the risk of heart disease, diabetes, stroke and cancer.

When you eliminate refined carbohydrates, you may experience some cravings, as your body is getting used to coming down from the blood-sugar roller coaster. However, the more you reduce your refined-carbohydrate intake, the less you will crave the stuff. You'll more than likely find that your appetite for this junk will diminish, and you have fewer blood-sugar swings, but more consistent energy. Your taste buds will also return to normal and you will start tasting food properly again.

Replace refined carbohydrate	*With*
White bread	Whole-grain or rye bread
Regular pasta	Wholewheat pasta
Ramen noodles	Buckwheat noodles
White rice	Brown rice
Concentrated fruit juice	Fruit
Breakfast cereals	Oatmeal

Sugar

Now let's look at the deadliest of all the refined carbohydrates – sugar.

The average person in the UK and Ireland now consumes up to 15 times more sugar than the average person 100 years ago. This amounts to almost 150 mgs of sugar per day. Most people do not have any idea that they are consuming so much as it is hidden in a wide variety of processed foods. But when you look more closely at what sugar actually does to your body's metabolism, you will start to wonder how the human body can continue to survive for as long as it does whilst consuming this deadly poison.

This huge increase in refined-sugar consumption has paralleled the dramatic rise in the incidence of heart disease. Heart disease at the beginning of the twentieth century was relatively rare. Now it accounts for almost half of all deaths. Scientific studies now indicate that sugar is a primary cause in this dramatic rise, as well as in the rise of other degenerative diseases, including cancer.

Knowing that there is such a strong link between sugar and life-challenging illnesses, you will understand that refined sugar must be avoided completely.

High sugar consumption has been shown to lead to chronically elevated insulin levels in the blood. Elevated insulin levels promote the formation of fat in the body and consequently increase the risk of heart attack. Those with the highest insulin levels in a Finnish study were three times as likely to have a heart attack as those with the lowest insulin levels. As high sugar consumption can also cause chronically elevated insulin levels, this suggests at least one reason why sugar is a strong factor in the causation of diabetes, a disease that in turn also increases the risk of heart disease.

When sugar enters your stomach it ferments, inhibiting your ability to digest and stopping the secretion of gastric juices. So drinking a soft drink with your meal causes the food to basically rot in your stomach.

When you give up sugar, there will be withdrawals at first as it is highly addictive, but very quickly your taste buds will awaken and everything will taste better and clearer. Food will come back to life again and start to taste like the good old days.

Ten Reasons to Avoid Sugar

1. Sugar can suppress your immune function and impair your defence against infectious disease.

2. Sugar upsets the mineral balance in your body, causing chromium and copper deficiency and interfering with the absorption of calcium and magnesium.

3. Sugar can produce a significant rise in total cholesterol, triglycerides and bad cholesterol and a decrease in good cholesterol, leading to a dramatically increased risk of heart disease.

4. Sugar can feed cancer cells, and studies have connected it with the development of cancers of the breast, ovaries, prostate, rectum, pancreas, biliary tract, lung, gall bladder and stomach.

5. Sugar can cause many gastrointestinal-tract problems, including indigestion, malabsorption in patients with functional bowel disease, increased risk of Crohn's disease and ulcerative colitis.

6. Sugar can impair your DNA structure.

7. Sugar intake is higher in people with Parkinson's disease.

8. Sugar can increase kidney size and contribute to the formation of kidney stones.

9. Diets high in sugar will increase free radicals, contributing to disease and oxidative stress.

10. Sugar can induce abnormal metabolic processes and promote chronic degenerative diseases.

Artificial Sweeteners – the Deadly Alternative

What about artificial sweeteners, such as aspartame (E951) and saccharine? The word 'artificial' should give you a hint. Steer clear of all man-made sweeteners as they have been linked with a wide variety of health problems. The FDA did not approve aspartame for 16 years because of concerns about its use. It has been linked to a variety of symptoms, including headaches, panic attacks, depression, seizures and, most frightening of all, multiple sclerosis and brain tumours. Aspartame is made from wood alcohol and saccharine is made from petroleum, and they are widely used in diet drinks and many junk foods. Unfortunately, they are also used in processed foods that are promoted as healthy options: you will see them in many low-fat yoghurts and desserts.

One reason why many people would choose aspartame or saccharine is because they wish to lose weight. However, a side effect of these sweeteners is that they elicit carbohydrate cravings, so the net result of using artificial sweeteners is that you tend to gain weight.

These artificial sweeteners also cause dehydration, which explains why only drinking a small amount of water quenches your thirst whilst you can drink a vast amount of a diet soft drink and still be thirsty.

All in all, there is no good reason to include artificial sweeteners in your diet and every reason to avoid them. An acceptable alternative to sugar is a moderate amount of organic honey and the natural sweetness you obtain from fruit.

Healthy Protein

Replace red and dark meat with healthier sources of protein.

The more we understand about nutrition and health, the more we realise that we should try to eat as low on the food chain as possible. Whilst we may harbour images of our ancestors hunting woolly mammoth, the truth is that we did not evolve by eating large quantities of red meat. Anthropological studies have now dismissed the concept of meat-eating cavemen. Throughout evolutionary history most of the human diet came from wild plants occasionally supplemented by small game and fish.

Humans are more herbivore than carnivore. Our closest living relatives in the animal world, apes, are 98% vegetarian. Our digestive systems have been designed to cater for a predominantly vegetarian diet.

Studies have shown a significantly increased risk of colon and prostate cancer in people who are heavy consumers of red meat. More specifically, it shows that the risk doubles compared to those who consume smaller quantities of red meat. But how does this compare to people who consume no red meat at all?

We used to think that the damage caused by red meat and the brown meat of pork was simply due to its saturated-fat content. It's true that the saturated fat found in red meat contributes to heart disease and atherosclerosis, but recent opinion is that this damage may have more to do with other factors. Research also shows that carcinogens are formed when meat is cooked, especially when it is well done, and this could be a direct cause of colon cancer.

In addition, meat products contain contaminants such as heavy metals, pesticides and various environmental pollutants that gather in the fat tissues of cows, which in turn are absorbed into our bodies when we eat the meat of that cow. This fat is pervasive throughout the meat even in the lean portions.

If more people knew about how meat was manufactured, the number of vegetarians would increase significantly. When the animal is killed, it gets a surge of adrenaline throughout its body. This adrenaline rush gets trapped in the flesh of the animal and that is what we eat when it arrives on our plate. The flesh we eat contains the animal's fear.

When eating the flesh of animal, you must consider another factor. Whatever that animal ate is ultimately going into your body. The food, the hormones, the toxins that have been given to that animal are ultimately yours if you eat its flesh. It is quite common for cows to be fed chicken litter, and those chickens were often fed diseased cows containing spinal-cord material that could carry mad-cow disease. Bearing this in mind, how much would that turn you off eating beef?

All these factors, together with the recent scares about *E. coli* and CJD, the human form of mad-cow disease, leave us in no doubt that our bodies are better off without the harmful effects of red meat.

Alternatives to Red and Dark Meat

The meats that are allowed as part of the Healing Code Nutrition Plan include oily fish, such as salmon, tuna and mackerel, and the white meat of organic free-range chicken and turkey. In addition to these meats, there are other far superior sources of protein that form the backbone of the Healing Code Nutrition Plan.

As discussed, oily fish provides omega-3 fatty acids, which are critical for maintaining the cardiovascular and the immune system. Fish is one of the best foods that you can eat for your heart. The omega-3 fat in fish is a platelet-inhibitor – it helps to prevent clots from forming in the coronary arteries and elsewhere. This fish oil will also help to lower bad cholesterol.

The white meat from organic free-range chicken and turkey is also a healthier alternative to red meat. It is lower in calories, lower in fat and higher in protein than red meat. Organically reared chicken and turkey must be chosen as these are raised without growth enhancements, on farms that do not use conventional pesticides, fertilisers, bioengineering methods or exposure to io-nising radiation. Products from these birds contain no artificial ingredients or preservatives and are minimally processed. When eating chicken or turkey, do remember to only eat the white meat, as it is the healthiest, and always remove the skin before cooking.

OK, so some of you reading this book will be vegetarian and will not want to eat meat at all. That's fine, however many vegetarians that come to my clinic actually have a very poor diet as they compensate for the lack of meat with overconsumption of dairy products. Make sure that you are abiding by the other principles of the Healing Code Nutrition Plan – avoid dairy products and ensure that you are getting adequate omega-3 from flaxseed or an alternative supplement.

You can also very healthily replace animal protein with vegetable protein and gain additional antioxidants, vitamins and minerals. Vegetarian meat substitutes are often made from soya. Numerous studies have shown that soya foods such as tofu can help to strengthen bones, reduce the risk of heart disease, breast cancer, prostate cancer and colon cancer. There is extensive research underway to formally document the real extent of the health benefits soybeans have on health. Scientists believe that isoflavones found in soybeans may actually inhibit the growth of cancer cells. Eating just 5 g of soya protein a day has been shown to lower blood cholesterol by 10%, and 40 g significantly increased bone density in the lumbar spine of postmenopausal women. Replacing animal protein with soya protein is therefore nutritionally sound, as soya contains all the essential amino acids needed to make human protein.

Nuts are also a good source of protein and provide excellent antioxidant benefits. Almonds and soya nuts are especially good, as they are high in heart-protecting monounsaturated fats. However, always avoid nuts that are salted.

Organic Fruit and Vegetables

Consume large quantities of organic fruit and vegetables.

'When I was 88 years old, I gave up meat entirely and switched to a plant-based diet, following a slight stroke. During the following months, I not only lost 50 lb but gained strength in my legs and picked up stamina. Now, at age 93, I'm on the same plant-based diet, and I still don't eat any meat or dairy products. I either swim, walk or paddle a canoe daily, and I feel the best I've felt since my heart problems began.' Benjamin Spock, MD

It is beyond any doubt that vegetables and fruit are really good for you. They are crammed full of nutrients, and we should generally aim for at least ten servings of fruit and vegetables a day. A diet high in fruit and vegetables significantly protects against heart disease, cancer, stroke and hypertension. Vegetables are one of the main sources of dietary antioxidants, and as discussed, this protects against cell damage and disease.

Whilst our bodies do have their own built-in immune system, our food supplies the protective ammunition. It therefore makes a lot of sense to load up on antioxidant-rich food rather than stocking up on empty calories. The most antioxidant-rich foods are fruit and vegetables.

No foods are more important for sustaining and recovering good health than fruit and vegetables. Gerson therapy has controversially asserted that these foods alone are enough to recover health from the most challenging of illnesses. Dr Max Gerson developed this therapy 60 years ago. It involves flooding the body with nutrients from about twenty pounds of organically grown fresh fruit and vegetables each day. A total of 13 glasses of juice are consumed daily, in addition to 3 regular meals. Coffee enemas are also used to intensify liver detoxification. Whilst the Healing Code Nutrition Plan doesn't go that far, organic fruit and vegetables are indeed the cornerstone of recovering health through nutrition. A recent survey conducted with 30,000 people living in the UK found that consumption of fruit and vegetables was positively correlated with *all* indicators of good health.

With the Healing Code Nutrition Plan, you will aim to eat *at least* ten portions of organic fruit and vegetables a day. A portion size is approximately the size of your fist. Remember that you are now in health-recovery mode so we are going to turbocharge your health with the most powerful nutrients. These nutrients are predominantly contained in fruit and vegetables and hence at least 80% of the food that you will eat should be plant-based.

The antioxidant level in your bloodstream determines a major component of your overall free-radical defence system. Although practically all fruit and vegetables contain almost pharmacological levels of antioxidants, some provide superior levels, which put them in the realm of superfoods.

A Note on Juicing

I have no doubt that juicing diets offer benefits. But the main reason why they work is because generally people are only juicing healthy antioxidant-rich foods. We don't juice burgers, chips, cake or sausages.

One of the main purposes of juicing is that it allows these powerful foods to be easily and rapidly digested. However, it is worth bearing in mind that some of the most important digestive enzymes occur in our mouths, supported by the salivary glands. If you eat properly, then there is absolutely no need to juice your food. The Chinese have a phrase 'You should drink your food and eat your drink', which means that you should spend time slowly chewing your food before you swallow it. The advantage of this approach over juicing is that some of the beneficial plant enzymes lost in the juicing process, particularly with lower-cost home juicers, remain in your body. Therefore, slowly masticating your food until it is almost liquefied gives you all the benefits of juicing and more. For most of us, this approach is also more pleasurable.

Water and Alcohol

Drink plenty of water and restrict alcohol consumption to a maximum of one glass of red wine per day.

You should not wait until you get thirsty until you drink water. Water is a major source of energy, and whilst we can survive many weeks without food, we can only survive a few days without water. By the time you get thirsty you have already become dehydrated. You have lost energy from the water you should have drunk before you got thirsty. You don't wait for your petrol tank to be empty before you refill it, so why wouldn't you treat your body with the same respect that you treat your car?

So, first thing, never allow yourself to get thirsty, and drink regularly throughout the day. You should drink at least two litres of water a day. Do try to stop drinking three hours before you retire for the evening. Sleep is also vitally important to your health recovery and drinking late in the evening can disturb sleep; however, if you are going to get dehydrated, always err on the side of water consumption.

When we drink water we are supporting our kidneys. When we drink enough water so that our urine is colourless, this is a good sign. When your urine is yellow, this is an early sign of dehydration. When it is orange, then you are truly dehydrated and some parts of your body are suffering as a result. This dehydration can manifest in exhaustion, depression and even pain.

Where we get our water from is the next thing to consider. Despite all the assurances given, unfiltered tap water is not a good source. Unfiltered tap water usually contains residues of harmful chemicals such as benzene, pesticides and disinfectant by-products. Chemicals seep into our water supplies from waste-disposal sites, as well as from pesticides that are swept into lakes and streams from land nearby.

I do not recommend mineral water either, as it often contains such high levels of radioactivity, nitrates and other pollutants that it would be illegal if it came out of a tap. A good approach is to filter your water through a standard charcoal filter, which will remove most of the harmful substances. You could also invest in a point-of-use filter, which you can locate at your kitchen sink and thereby treat all the water that you use in the kitchen.

After filtering, it's a good idea to then boil the water and drink it warm, as this is more beneficial to digestion. Cold water is considered by Chinese medicine to put a strain on your digestive system, as your body has to work hard to heat it up. Therefore avoid drinking water direct from the fridge, and bear in mind that warm water combats dehydration just as well as cold water.

What about soft drinks? Well, most soft drinks contain refined carbohydrates, which, as discussed, have a hugely detrimental effect on our bodies. But apart from this, soft drinks do not provide the same level of hydration as water. As soft drinks contain vast amounts of sugar and phosphates, they also have a dehydrating effect and can cause the excretion of more water than they provide, resulting in a net loss of water and *not* a net gain.

What about alcohol? Alcohol rapidly dehydrates your body. When you are hung-over you are actually suffering from the effects of dehydration. This is why a good hangover prevention is to drink a lot of water after you have had a lot of alcohol. There is very little positive that can be said for alcohol in terms of your health.

The French Paradox

The one exception is red wine. The protective qualities of red wine have led to what has become known as the 'French Paradox'. Although the French eat as much saturated fat as the British or Irish, they have much healthier hearts. It is worth noting that we are only talking about red wine. Recent studies have shown a close relationship between moderate drinking of red wine and a healthy heart. Moderation usually means one glass of red wine a day. White wine and other forms of alcohol do not have the same benefits and are generally considered harmful. Using a small amount infrequently in cooking is, however, acceptable.

The beneficial effect of red wine is still not fully understood, but is thought to be partly due to the high antioxidant levels, which protect the walls of blood vessels, helping to maintain their normal permeability and also protecting blood cholesterol from harmful oxidation. Scientists from Harvard Medical School also believe that a key molecule, resveratrol, which is found in abundance in red wine, gives it its anticancer and anti-heart-disease properties. Research has suggested that daily consumption of a single glass of red wine gives 13% protection against cancer when compared with non-drinkers.

Coffee and Tea – the Alternatives

Replace coffee and tea with green and jasmine tea.

Caffeine is technically an insecticide, as are morphine and cocaine. They are from the same family of drugs and are neurotoxins. In other words, they are harmful to the nervous system. Most people get caffeine from coffee or tea. Caffeine is also a powerful diuretic, which means it robs your body of much-needed water and places strain on your kidneys and liver.

- Caffeine affects the central nervous system, the brain, lungs, heart, muscles and digestive system, raises blood pressure, increases heart rate and calms the smooth muscles.
- Caffeine increases the release of adrenaline and can raise anxiety levels and cause panic.
- Caffeine increases the amount of calcium excreted in your urine.
- Caffeine causes insomnia.
- Caffeine can cause gastrointestinal upsets including constipation and diarrhoea.

- Caffeine increases stomach-acid secretion. The stomach acids back up into the oesophagus and produce heartburn.
- Caffeine reduces iron absorption.

The other problem with caffeine is that it sends you into a vicious circle. As caffeine is a stimulant, it affects sleeping patterns, which in turn will adversely affect your health recovery. Deprived of sleep, you then feel it necessary to drink more caffeine just to keep yourself awake. This caffeine roller coaster does little to support your health recovery. Coffee lowers blood sugar and stems the flow of blood to the brain. This can cause palpitations and anxiety. You should avoid taking decaffeinated coffee, as it contains other harmful chemicals such as turpentine and formaldehyde.

Green tea and jasmine tea are excellent choices as a substitute for tea or coffee. Although green and jasmine teas do contain caffeine, the levels are substantially lower than those found in coffee and other teas. The substantial health benefits associated with green and jasmine teas therefore overwhelmingly outweigh any negative effect associated with this minimal amount of caffeine. Drinking green tea after a meal is considered an excellent aid to digestion. Scientific research in both Asia and the West is providing hard evidence for the health benefits long associated with drinking green tea. In 1994 the *Journal of the National Cancer Institute* published the results of an epidemiological study indicating that drinking green tea reduced the risk of oesophageal cancer in men and women by nearly 60%. University of Purdue researchers recently concluded that a compound in green tea inhibits the growth of cancer cells. There is also research indicating that drinking green tea improves the ratio of good to bad cholesterol.

Jasmine tea contains all the goodness of green tea and more. It is made from green tea leaves combined with fresh jasmine flowers. Research studies have shown that laboratory animals live up 20% longer when jasmine tea was added to drinking water. The winning components of jasmine tea are the artery-cleansing flavonoids and the high antioxidant levels. Many studies have shown the potential role of tea flavonoids in cancer prevention, including cancers of the lung, breast, prostate, bladder, stomach and colon. They have also been shown to be effective in helping to prevent heart disease and stroke.

It is worth noting that we are talking about green tea and jasmine tea as opposed to plain old breakfast tea. The principal difference is that these teas have not been oxidised and therefore have retained the quantity of flavonoids that helps to reap the health benefits. You should therefore drink up to three cups of green or jasmine tea per day and avoid coffee and regular tea.

Table Salt

> Replace refined table salt with healthy spices.

Whilst salt is necessary for proper body function, it also contributes to a variety of health problems when consumed in excess. It is considered that only 500 mg of dietary sodium meets our body's daily needs. You can fulfil this by following the Healing Code Nutrition Plan without adding any table salt or other forms of sodium.

An average person consumes 15 times the required daily amount of dietary sodium, which can lead to hypertension, cause calcium, magnesium and potassium deficiencies as well as heart attacks, strokes, kidney failure and a myriad of other conditions.

Too much salt has been proven by scientists in the University of Sydney to have a dangerous adrenaline-inducing effect on people suffering from hypertension. When we get a fright, our nervous systems get a rush of adrenaline, but those with high blood pressure who consume refined salt experience a sustained increase in sympathetic nerve activity. They are left in a continuous state of heightened stress otherwise known as the 'fight or flight' response, which can last for months or even years. For more information on the 'fight or flight' response, turn to page 76.)

In addition to the salt we add to our food, many foods contain sodium as a part of their normal chemical composition. Ingredients such as baking powder, baking soda, soy sauce, pickles and olives contain significant amounts of sodium. Many processed foods also contain added sodium. The chemical additives contained in processed foods contain large amounts of sodium – monosodium glutamate, sodium phosphate, sodium nitrite and sodium benzoate, to name but a few.

With the Healing Code Nutrition Plan you will therefore stop using table salt. As you will be avoiding processed foods, you will simply get adequate sodium from natural sources. If you wish to season food to add taste, you can add any of the following healthy alternatives: basil, bay leaves, cayenne, cinnamon, cloves, cumin, curry leaf, dill seeds, fennel, garlic, ginger, horseradish, mustard seeds, paprika, parsley, pepper, saffron, sesame seeds, Szechuan pepper, tamarind, thyme and turmeric.

The Healing Code Supplements

A significant element of empowering your body for healing is in making sure that your vitamin intake is adequate. A number of vitamins are required in small amounts for good nutrition. These consist of fat-soluble vitamins A, D, E and K, the water-soluble B vitamins and vitamin C. Most processed foods are depleted of vitamins, and this often results in our bodies being starved of these vital nutrients. Vitamin deficiency results in a number of symptoms, such as fatigue, weakness, loss of appetite and so forth. Vitamin A deficiency is associated with eye problems such as dry eyes and even blindness. Vitamin B is particularly important for carbohydrate metabolism. Severe vitamin B deficiency results in symptoms such as mental confusion and paralysis, and even heart failure can occur. Vitamin C deficiency can lead to very poor healing recovery after injury and lowered immunity.

The earth's soils have become increasingly depleted in a number of vital nutrients, and as a result, plants are often lacking in a variety of essential nutrients. Whilst chemical fertilisers can cause toxic harm to our bodies, they can also be effective at stimulating crop growth within these nutrient-poor soils. This results in the soils becoming progressively depleted even though the crops continue to grow. Though the resultant vegetables appear to prosper, they are lacking in the full range of minerals and vitamins.

The best way to attain vitamins is through a high-quality and varied organic diet, as recommended by the Healing Code Nutrition Plan. However, I also recommend that you supplement your diet with the following vitamins and minerals as there is gathering scientific evidence that they lend support in fighting many serious illnesses.

The following supplement programme is therefore part of the Healing Code Nutrition Plan:

Supplement	Daily Dosage
Spirulina	6,000 mg
Vitamin A (contained in spirulina)	15,000 IU
Vitamin B complex	50 mg
Vitamin C	2,000–10,000 mg
Vitamin E	1,000 mg
Zinc	30 mg
Selenium	200 mcg
Coenzyme Q10	400 mg
MSM	2,000 mg

Spirulina

Spirulina is the most nutritious concentrated food – animal or plant – known to man, delivering many nutrients that are lacking in most people's diets. It is the richest whole-food source of beta carotene (vitamin A) and is 25 times richer than raw carrots in beta carotene. Beta carotene is a natural antioxidant that offers powerful protection against free-radical damage.

Spirulina is also the richest whole-food source of vitamin B12, which provides energy and is essential for normal growth and neurological function.

According to a study by Prof. Hiroshi Nagamura from Tokai University, Japan, the gamma linolenic acid (GLA) from spirulina can substantially help to lower cholesterol levels in the blood. Moreover, the research reported that vitamins and minerals in spirulina can be more readily absorbed into the bloodstream than those found in meat. GLA is a fatty acid that supports normal blood pressure, proper joint function, reduces premenstrual stress and improves skin health.

Spirulina has twice the protein level of its nearest rival, the soybean, and at least three times that of beef, fish or eggs. The protein make-up of spirulina has a superior complete amino-acid profile: it contains all eight essential amino acids and ten non-essential amino acids in the correct proportions. It is the most digestible form of protein, and the amino acids in spirulina are delivered in an essentially 'free-form' state for almost instantaneous assimilation.

Spirulina helps protect the immune system, reduce cholesterol and aid in the absorption of minerals. It has been used in the treatment of diabetes, glaucoma, liver pathologies and cancer. For those with hypoglycaemia, a spirulina supplement can help regulate blood sugar levels between meals.

Dosage: 6,000 mg per day.

Research at the Osaka Institute of Public Health in Japan has shown that spirulina promotes the activation of natural cancer-fighting substances in the body.

In this clinical study, volunteers over 40 years of age were given 50 ml of a spirulina extract and the level of natural cancer-fighting substances were measured in their blood. The results showed that spirulina significantly increased the tumour-killing ability of natural killer cells and interferon gamma. The cell activity was increased one to two weeks after administration of spirulina. Furthermore, the activity continued for a surprising 12–24 weeks even after stopping the administration of spirulina.

Vitamin A (Beta Carotene)

Beta carotene helps prevent night blindness, other eye problems and skin disorders. It enhances immunity and protects against toxins, colds and flu. It is an antioxidant and protector of the cells and helps to slow the ageing process. Vitamin A also helps fight against both viral and bacterial infections.

Vitamin A deficiency has been associated with cancer occurrence and progression. A number of studies have found that beta carotene supplements increase the activity of natural killer cells and consequently help to protect against cancer. New research has shown that beta carotene not only helps prevent cancer but also helps to fight it.

If you are pregnant, do not take more than 6,000 IU of vitamin A, as higher doses have been associated with birth defects.

Research in China has shown that supplementation with vitamin A, combined with vitamin E and selenium substantially decreased cancer incidence. Beta carotene in the body can actually change into a substance called retinoic acid, now used to treat cancer.

Dosage: 15,000 IU per day – contained in spirulina.

Vitamin B

The B vitamins, collectively known as B complex, promote healthy nerves, skin, eyes, hair, liver, gastrointestinal tract and brain function. The B-complex vitamins work together as a team and help support healthy heart function, enhance and stimulate the immune system and inhibit the growth of cancerous cells and tumours. The B vitamins are also coenzymes involved in energy production. B complex is important for elderly people, and a deficiency can mimic Alzheimer's disease.

A team of American and Chinese researchers has discovered that vitamin B9 (folic acid) is highly effective in preventing breast cancer in women. The researchers found a clear correlation between dietary intake of folic acid and the risk of breast cancer.

It's also estimated that individuals with low vitamin B6 levels have a five times greater risk of having a heart attack than individuals with higher B6 levels.

B-complex vitamins help in the treatment of numerous health conditions, including ADHD, Alzheimer's disease, Crohn's disease, anxiety, depression, fatigue, diabetes, epilepsy, canker sores, heart disease, infertility, multiple sclerosis, rosacea, psoriasis and more. **Dosage: 50 mg.**

Vitamin C (Ascorbic Acid)

The famous two-time Nobel laureate Linus Pauling, PhD, did much to reveal vitamin C's powerful healing potential. He believed that as many as 75% of all cancer fatalities could be avoided through proper use of vitamin C. Vitamin C is one of the most potent antioxidants known to science and is a powerful free-radical scavenger. It protects against abnormal cells and prevents the destruction of DNA. It also stimulates the production of interferon, a powerful anticancer agent.

Vitamin C, or ascorbic acid, assists iron and calcium absorption, fights infection and plays an essential role in the immune system. Vitamin C reduces cholesterol and high blood pressure to prevent arteriosclerosis. It is very important for the growth and repair of body-tissue cells, gums, blood vessels, teeth and bones. It is found in every cell of our body and performs various functions.

One of the questions about vitamin C is how much of it you should take. Dr Pauling himself recommended 10,000 mg per day. It is perfectly safe to take high doses of vitamin C, as your body will naturally excrete any excess. However, if you do take a high dosage, you will need to build this level up over the course of a week or two, as taking high doses of vitamin C can lead to diarrhoea. Should this occur, reduce your dosage by half and gradually build back up. **Dosage: 2,000–10,000 mg per day.**

Vitamin E

Vitamin E is a fat-soluble vitamin of critical importance in the prevention of a number of medical conditions, including cancer, cardiovascular disease, diabetes, arthritis, cataracts and ageing. Vitamin E is a potent antioxidant and has a powerful effect on the brain. Vitamin E also protects us against free radicals and wards off heart disease. It causes dilation of the blood vessels, permitting a fuller flow of blood to the heart. Vitamin E inhibits coagulation of the blood, preventing clots from forming.

Vitamin E has been shown to fight cancer cells without affecting normal cells during radiation therapy. When combined with vitamin C and selenium, it helps to reduce the growth of breast- and prostate-cancer cells.

Dosage: 1,000 mg per day.

Observational studies have associated lower rates of heart disease with high vitamin E intake. A study of approximately ninety thousand nurses suggested that the incidence of heart disease was 30% to 40% lower among nurses with the highest intake of vitamin E from diet and supplements.

Zinc

Zinc is an essential mineral and plays an important role in prostate-gland function, as well as in the growth and health of the reproductive organs. This mineral is required for the synthesis of protein and the formation of collagen, and also plays an important part in promoting a healthy immune system and in healing wounds.

Zinc is involved in the body's ability to taste and smell and protects the liver from chemical damage. It is also vital for bone formation, as well as being a constituent of insulin and many important enzymes.

Zinc is a powerful antioxidant, and an adequate intake of zinc is required to assist the body's use of vitamin E in the blood. This mineral also has synergy with many other vitamins, assisting their absorption into the body.

Dosage: 30 mg per day.

Selenium

Selenium is a nutrient that plays a critical role in the production of antioxidant enzymes that protect cells against the effects of free radicals, which are produced during normal oxygen metabolism. Selenium is therefore essential for normal functioning of the immune system. Free radicals can damage cells and contribute to the development of some chronic diseases, such as Benign protastic hyperplasia (BPH) and prostate cancer.

This naturally occurring trace mineral protects your body against free radicals generated by smoke, pollution, radiation and other environmental toxins. Selenium also helps maintain healthy muscles. Selenium aids in the production of antibodies and helps maintain a healthy heart and liver, and when combined with vitamin E and zinc, it helps provide relief from an enlarged prostate. Studies have shown some positive effects of selenium when used in the treatment of arthritis, cardiovascular disease, male infertility, AIDS and high blood pressure. Further scientific studies have shown that selenium inhibits the growth of tumours, and there is some evidence that AIDS patients also have benefited when they take a selenium supplement as it increases red and white blood cell counts.

Its other benefits include being involved with iodine metabolism, pancreatic function, DNA repair, immunity and the detoxification of heavy metals.

Dosage: 200 mcg per day.

Coenzyme Q10

Imagine each cell in your body is a tiny engine. This engine uses oxygen to burn the fuels that come from food. CoQ10 is part of the engine that provides the 'spark' for this process. No other substance will substitute for CoQ10. Without CoQ10, there is no spark and therefore no production of energy.

Research studies have demonstrated the health benefits of taking CoQ10, some of which are improved cardiovascular function and blood circulation, increased energy levels and less fatigue, lowered blood pressure, reduced angina, and it is a strong anti-oxidant and anti-ageing nutrient. Coenzyme Q10 may also help prevent or slow Alzheimer's and Parkinson's disease.

CoQ10 is found in all food but is easily destroyed by cooking. Most people don't get enough dietary CoQ10. Your liver can also produce CoQ10 through a complex process requiring the presence of a large number of co-factors and three different classes of starting molecules. The benefits of CoQ10 to the heart and cardiovascular system have been extensively documented. People with poor heart-muscle contraction benefit greatly from CoQ10 as it increases heart contraction strength and boosts health recovery. It has also been shown that CoQ10 can aid in the full or partial remission of breast tumours as well as retarding tumour growth in general. There are over three hundred published papers on the disease-preventing roles of CoQ10.

Dosage: 400 mg per day.

MSM

Methyl-sulfonyl-methane (MSM) is a natural form of organic sulphur that is present in low concentrations throughout our body's tissues. Many foods contain MSM, but it is rapidly depleted during the cooking process. MSM helps maintain healthy cells and is a supplement that is generally supportive of good immune function.

You cannot overdose with MSM. The body will use what it needs and after 12 hours will flush any excess out of the body, and because it is a free radical and foreign-protein scavenger, MSM cleans the bloodstream, so relieves allergies to food and pollens. To maintain good, healthy cells, take MSM in the morning and evening.

Dosage: 2,000 mg.

Chinese Herbal Medicine

Herbal medicine is a major pillar of oriental medicine. Chinese herbal formulae are made from the roots, stems, bark, leaves or flowers of many plants, as well as some mineral and animal products. They are taken by over one billion people in Asia and have been used for thousands of years.

There are over four hundred herbs in use today. Chinese herbs are usually prescribed as a carefully balanced combination. The preparation and combining of the herbs requires considerable experience. Many of the herb combinations are therefore prepared and imported from China. Specific combinations of herbs may be useful as tonics for people who are depleted in energy and may be used to treat a wide variety of conditions.

Chinese herbal medicine also involves dietary therapy, as proper nutrition is seen as fundamental to maintaining optimum health, as well as for the treatment of disease. Foods have many similar properties to herbs, and an old Chinese adage asks, 'Are herbs food, or food herbs?'

Chinese herbs cure energetically by stimulating energy flow in the meridians. Different herbs enter different channels and affect different internal organs. Chinese herbal medicine is a comprehensive form of medicine that can effectively address a wide variety of conditions. It has a long clinical history of treating acute and chronic conditions and often excels in treating conditions that Western medicine has difficulty in treating, as well as conditions that often go undiagnosed in Western medicine, such as chronic fatigue and IBS.

In order to get Chinese herbal medicine prescribed that is appropriate to your condition, you will need to visit a qualified and registered Chinese medical practitioner. As part of your recovery programme, I highly recommend that you do this.

If you are interested in finding out more about Chinese herbal medicine, contact one of the following organisations:

UK
The British Acupuncture Council (BAcC)
63 Jeddo Road
London W12 9HQ
Tel: 020 8735 0400 Fax: 020 8735 0404
Email: info@acupuncture.org.uk

Ireland
Traditional Chinese Medicine Council of Ireland
Station House
Sandyford
Dublin 18

Tel: 1850 300 600
Email: info@tcmci.ie

The Healing Code Menu

Breakfast

Oriental Mushroom Omelette
Scrambled Onion and Tofu
Poached Pear and Porridge
Strawberry and Banana Soya Milkshake
Chicken and Vegetable Stir-fry

Lunch

Chicken and Lentil Soup
Sweet Potato and Onion Soup
Tuna and Spinach Salad
Tofu Stir-fry with Oriental Vegetables
Chicken Teriyaki Stir-fry
Carrot and Green Bean Salad

Green tea after lunch

Dinner

Courgette and Carrot Stir-fry
Spicy Tofu
Black Bean Stir-fry
Chilli Bean Bake
Plaice Provençal

Salmon Pilaff
Monkfish Skewers
Grilled Chicken Salsa
Chicken, Pineapple and Ginger Stir-fry

Green tea after dinner

Dessert

Cherry Baked Apples
Mixed Berry and Fruit Salad

Snack Options

Any of the immuno-conditioned (or healing) foods listed on page 58
Fresh fruit
Dried fruit
Nut mix (unsalted)

For further menu options, please consult www.healing-code.com.

Breakfast Recipes

Oriental Mushroom Omelette

organic extra-virgin olive oil
2 eggs, lightly beaten
freshly ground black pepper
50 g (2 oz) fresh spinach
75 g (3 oz) fresh shiitake/oyster mushrooms, sliced
ground paprika

Serves one

Coat the frying pan with extra-virgin olive oil and preheat over a
medium-low heat. Place the eggs in the pan and sprinkle with the
pepper. Let the eggs cook without stirring for about two minutes,
or until set around the edges. Use a spatula to lift the edges of the
omelette and allow the uncooked egg to flow below the cooked

portion. Cook for another minute or two, until the eggs are almost set. Arrange the spinach and the mushrooms over half of the omelette. Fold the other half over the filling and cook for another minute or two, or until the eggs are completely set. Slide the omelette on to a plate, sprinkle with paprika and serve immediately.

Scrambled Onion and Tofu

1 small onion, finely chopped
organic extra-virgin olive oil
150 g (5 oz) plain silken tofu
1 clove of garlic
¼ tsp dried dill
freshly ground black pepper
Tabasco

Serves one to two

Using a frying pan, gently sauté the onion in a little extra-virgin olive oil until softened but not browned. Add the tofu and stir-fry for about another ten minutes. Crush the garlic together with the dill and add a few tablespoons of water. Season the tofu with ground black pepper and a splash of Tabasco. Add the garlic and dill to the pan. Stir and cook until the liquid is gone and the scrambled tofu is fairly dry. Serve immediately.

Poached Pear and Porridge

100 g (3½ oz) porridge oats
2 fresh pears, pitted and halved
2 tbsp raw honey
1 tbsp lemon juice
low-fat organic soya milk

Serves one

Soak the oats in 360 ml (12 fl oz) of boiling water for about ten minutes. Put the pears in a saucepan with the honey and lemon juice and two tablespoons of water and simmer for about ten minutes until the pears are soft. Serve the porridge with the pears and add low-fat organic soya milk.

Strawberry and Banana Soya Milkshake

150 g (5 oz) strawberries
240 ml (8 fl oz) organic soya milk
1 mashed banana

Serves one

Blend all the ingredients (reserving a small piece of banana) very well, preferably in a household mixer. Serve in a wine glass, garnished with the piece of banana.

Chicken and Vegetable Stir-fry

1 tbsp soy sauce
1 tsp fresh ginger
2 cloves of garlic, crushed
organic extra-virgin olive oil
450 g (1 lb) organic chicken breast, diced
3 tbsp organic low-sodium vegetable stock
3 tsp organic oyster sauce
1 tsp cornflour
1 onion, diced
150 g (5 oz) mangetout
250 g (9 oz) bok choy, chopped
150 g (5 oz) baby corn
4 tbsp coriander leaves, chopped
2 spring onions, chopped
brown rice (cooked beforehand)

Serves four

For those used to eating a hearty breakfast, there is no reason to stop now. However, rather than a fry-up, try this delicious alternative.

Mix together the soy sauce, ginger, garlic and the extra-virgin olive oil in a non-metallic bowl. Add the chicken and stir in well. Cover and marinate in the fridge for two hours.

In a separate bowl, mix the stock and oyster sauce together with the cornflour. Heat a wok and add some extra-virgin olive oil. Add the marinated chicken and stir-fry until just cooked through. Remove from the wok. Heat more oil in the wok and add the onion. Stir-fry for two to three minutes, then add the mangetout, bok choy and baby corn. Stir-fry for a further three minutes. Add the stir-fry sauce (the cornflour mixture) and the chicken, along with any juices. Stir well and cook for about three minutes, or until the sauce has thickened to lightly coat the chicken and vegetables. Remove from the heat and stir in the coriander and spring onion. Season and serve with the pre-prepared brown rice.

Lunch Recipes

Chicken and Lentil Soup

2 tbsp organic extra-virgin olive oil
1 carrot, chopped
1 onion, chopped
2 sticks of celery, chopped
3 tbsp dry white wine
700 ml (24 fl oz) organic low-sodium chicken stock
2 tsp dried thyme
1 bay leaf
150 g (5 oz) red or green lentils
225 g (8 oz) cooked organic free-range chicken breast, diced
freshly ground black pepper

Serves four

Pour the extra-virgin olive oil into a large saucepan. Add the carrot, onion and celery. Cook for three to five minutes, until softened. Stir in the wine and the chicken stock. Bring to the boil and skim off any surface foam. Add the thyme and bay leaf. Reduce the heat, cover and simmer for 30 minutes. Add the lentils and continue cooking, covered, for another 30–40 minutes, until they are just tender, stirring the soup from time to time. Stir in the diced chicken and season to taste with the pepper. Cook until just heated through. Pour the soup into bowls and serve hot.

Sweet Potato and Onion Soup

1 kg (2 lb 2 oz) sweet potatoes, peeled
2 onions, peeled and halved
1 litre (33 fl oz) organic low-sodium chicken stock
1 tbsp fresh thyme, chopped, plus 1 tsp thyme leaves
1 tsp curry powder
pinch of cayenne
freshly ground black pepper

Serves four

Preheat the oven to 425°F (220°C). Put the sweet potatoes and the onion halves on a baking tray. Roast the vegetables until they are soft when pierced with a large fork. Cut the potatoes and onions into large chunks and put in a food processor. Purée with half the chicken stock. Transfer to a large pot. Whisk in the remaining stock. Add the thyme, curry and cayenne. Bring to the boil and then simmer for 20 minutes. Season with pepper and fresh thyme leaves.

Tuna and Spinach Salad

125 g (4 oz) spinach leaves
375 g (13 oz) kidney beans (cooked beforehand)
375 g (13 oz) tuna (cooked beforehand)
1 cucumber, thinly sliced
2 tomatoes, diced
2 tbsp parsley, chopped
2 tbsp extra-virgin olive oil

2 tbsp lemon juice
freshly ground black pepper

Serves four

Divide the spinach, pre-prepared kidney beans, tuna, cucumber, tomato and parsley between four plates. Combine the oil, lemon juice and pepper, and pour over the salads.

Tofu Stir-fry with Oriental Vegetables

500 g (1 lb 2 oz) tofu
4 tbsp organic extra-virgin olive oil
400 g (14 oz) shiitake mushrooms, sliced
150 g (5 oz) mangetout
2 cloves of garlic, finely chopped
2 tomatoes, sliced
3 tbsp soy sauce
1 tsp thyme
freshly ground black pepper

Serves four

Cut the tofu into cubes. Heat some extra-virgin olive oil in a wok and stir-fry the tofu for two or three minutes until golden brown. Take the tofu out, drain and keep warm.

Warm the remaining oil in the wok and add the sliced mushroom, mangetout, garlic, tomatoes, soy sauce and 240 ml of water. Stir-fry for two minutes.

Put the tofu cubes back in the wok and stir gently. Add the thyme. Season with freshly ground black pepper and serve.

Chicken Teriyaki Stir-fry

4 organic free-range chicken breasts
organic extra-virgin olive oil
3 tbsp organic teriyaki sauce
1 onion, chopped

75 g (3 oz) mushrooms, sliced
½ head cabbage, chopped
10 broccoli florets
100 g (3½ oz) snow peas
1 red pepper, deseeded and chopped
brown rice (cooked beforehand)

Serves four

Cut the chicken into bite-size strips and cook in a wok in a little extra-virgin olive oil. When the chicken is almost finished cooking, add a teaspoon of the teriyaki sauce. Let it finish cooking, stirring occasionally so it doesn't burn. Remove the cooked chicken from the wok and set aside. Sauté the onions and mushrooms with about two teaspoons of extra-virgin olive oil and add the chopped cabbage.

In a separate pot, steam the broccoli. When the cabbage is nearly done, add the chicken and broccoli to the wok. Add the rest of the teriyaki sauce, the snow peas and the red pepper. Simmer until everything is hot. Serve with brown rice.

Carrot and Green Bean Salad

450 g (1 lb) green beans, sliced lengthwise
4 carrots, thinly sliced
3 tbsp vinegar
3 tbsp organic extra-virgin olive oil
2 onions, thinly sliced
1 red pepper, deseeded and thinly sliced
1 tsp dried dill seeds
freshly ground black pepper

Serves four

Cook the sliced beans and carrots in boiling water until just tender. Drain the vegetables and create stock using 60 ml (2 fl oz) of the water that the green beans and carrots were cooked in. Transfer them to a large salad bowl.

Prepare the dressing by combining the vinegar, oil, the vegetable wait until it cools stock, onions, red pepper and dill seeds. Stir until blended. Pour the mixture over the beans and marinate for several hours. Season with ground black pepper and serve.

Dinner

Courgette and Carrot Stir-fry

250 g (9 oz) carrots
3 courgettes
3 tbsp organic extra-virgin olive oil
3 cloves of garlic, crushed
freshly ground black pepper

Serves four

Cut carrots julienne style (two- to three-inch-long strips). Peel the courgettes and cut into strips. Heat the olive oil over a medium heat. Add the carrots and stir-fry for two minutes. Add the crushed garlic and the courgettes. Stir-fry for a further four minutes. Lower the heat, season, stir and serve.

Spicy Tofu

500 g (1 lb 2 oz) soft tofu
1 tbsp extra-virgin olive oil
1 tbsp ginger, finely chopped
1 clove of garlic, crushed
1 tbsp organic chilli-bean sauce
1 tbsp organic yellow-bean sauce
¼ tbsp organic low-sodium vegetable stock
2 tbsp dry sherry
1 tsp cornflour
2 tbsp spring onions, chopped
brown rice (cooked beforehand)

Serves four

Cut the tofu into one-inch cubes. Heat a wok over a high heat, adding the extra-virgin olive oil. Put in the ginger, garlic, chilli-bean sauce and yellow-bean sauce, and stir-fry for 30 seconds.

Add the stock and sherry, and cook for two minutes. Mix the cornflour with a teaspoon of water and add to the wok.

After the sauce has slightly thickened, add the tofu cubes and stir gently. Continue to cook for two minutes until the tofu is heated thoroughly. Garnish with the chopped spring onions and serve at once with brown rice.

Black Bean Stir-fry

2 tbsp extra-virgin olive oil
2 tbsp fresh ginger, crushed
1 yellow pepper, deseeded and chopped
450 g (1 lb) mixed vegetables, chopped
225 g (8 oz) black beans
3 tbsp tamari
3 tbsp rice vinegar
brown rice (cooked beforehand)

Serves four

Heat the oil in a wok and add the ginger. Sauté for approximately one minute until fragrant. Add the yellow pepper and other vegetables. Cover and sauté for about five minutes until slightly soft. Add the black beans, tamari and rice vinegar. Stir-fry for another few minutes. Serve over brown rice.

Chilli Bean Bake

225 g (8 oz) red kidney beans
1 bay leaf
1 large onion, chopped
1 clove of garlic, crushed
1 tsp chilli powder
2 celery sticks, diced

450 g (1 lb) tomatoes, chopped
1 tsp dried mixed herbs
1 tbsp lemon juice
1 yellow pepper, deseeded and diced
1 tsp cumin

Serves four

Leave the beans to soak overnight in cold water. Drain and rinse well.

Preheat the oven to 425°F (220°C). Pour a litre of water into a large saucepan and add the beans and bay leaf. Boil for ten minutes. Simmer for 40 minutes until the beans are tender.

Add the onion, garlic, chilli powder, celery, tomatoes and dried mixed herbs. Cover the pan and simmer for another ten minutes. Stir in the lemon juice, yellow pepper and cumin. Simmer for another ten minutes, stirring until the vegetables are tender. Remove the bay leaf and transfer the mixture into a large casserole dish. Bake in the oven for 20 minutes.

Plaice Provençal

2 red onions
240 ml (8 fl oz) organic vegetable stock
4 tbsp red wine
1 clove of garlic, crushed
1 yellow pepper, deseeded and sliced
8 tomatoes, chopped
1 tbsp fresh thyme, chopped
freshly ground black pepper
4 fillets of fresh plaice
brown rice (cooked beforehand)

Serves four

Preheat the oven to 350°F (180°C). Cut each onion into eight wedges and put into a saucepan with the stock. Cover and simmer for five minutes. Uncover and continue to cook, stirring occasionally, until the stock has reduced entirely. Add the wine and garlic to the pan and cook until the onions are soft. Add the yellow pepper, tomatoes and thyme and season to taste. Simmer for three minutes. Spoon the sauce into a large casserole. Fold each fillet in half and put on top of the sauce. Cover and cook in the oven for 15–20 minutes. Serve immediately with the pre-prepared brown rice.

Salmon Pilaff

1 red onion, chopped
5 celery sticks, chopped
1 red pepper, deseeded and diced
225 g (8 oz) brown rice
600ml (20 fl oz) organic fish stock
1 clove of garlic, crushed
1 medium glass white wine
450 g (1 lb) organic pink salmon
450 g (1 lb) kidney beans, soaked overnight
8 broccoli florets
2 tbsp fresh parsley, chopped
2 tbsp soy sauce
freshly ground black pepper
toasted flaked almonds to garnish

Serves four

Place the onion, celery, red pepper, rice, stock, garlic and wine in a saucepan. Stir and bring to the boil. Simmer for 25–30 minutes, until almost all the liquid has been absorbed, stirring occasionally.

Stir the salmon and kidney beans into the mixture, cooking gently for a further five to ten minutes. Meanwhile, cook the broccoli in boiling water for about five minutes, keeping it crispy. Transfer the broccoli gently into the pilaff. Stir in the parsley and soy sauce, and season to taste. Garnish with the toasted flaked almonds and serve immediately whilst hot.

Monkfish Skewers

2 tbsp fresh ginger
3 lemons
1 kg (2 lb 2oz) monkfish
4 onions, cut into quarters
2 egg whites
4 tbsp cornflour
extra-virgin olive oil
freshly ground black pepper

Serves four

Peel and chop the ginger and place in a bowl. Add the juice of two of the lemons and mix. Dice the monkfish and marinate with the lemon juice in the fridge for one hour, turning occasionally. Drain the monkfish and thread the pieces on bamboo skewers, alternating with onion quarters. Beat the egg whites using a fork in a small bowl, adding the cornflour. Dip the skewers in the mix. Fry the skewers in a pan for two to three minutes in extra-virgin olive oil. Drain, and serve immediately with lemon quarters season with ground pepper.

Grilled Chicken Salsa

4 organic free-range chicken breasts
2 tbsp organic extra-virgin olive oil
450 g (1 lb) watermelon
1 red onion
1 green chilli
5 tbsp coriander, chopped
2 tbsp lime juice
freshly ground black pepper

Serves four

Preheat the grill to medium. Brush the chicken with extra-virgin olive oil and grill for 15–20 minutes. To make the salsa, remove the skin and seeds from the watermelon. Dice and place into a bowl.

Chop the onion and chilli (removing the seeds) and mix with the melon. Add the coriander and lime juice, and season with black pepper. Pour the salsa into a small bowl. Serve the chicken on individual plates garnished with the salsa mix.

Chicken, Pineapple and Ginger Stir-fry

2 organic free-range chicken breasts, diced
2 cloves of garlic, crushed
2 tbsp ginger, thinly sliced
3 tbsp organic extra-virgin olive oil
1 pineapple, diced
2 carrots, sliced
1 green pepper, deseeded and sliced
60 ml (2 fl oz) pineapple juice
1 tbsp cornflour
20 ml (4 fl oz) soy sauce
3 onions, chopped
brown rice (cooked beforehand)

Serves four

Stir-fry the chicken, garlic and ginger in a wok with the extra-virgin olive oil for two minutes. Add the pineapple, carrots and green pepper. Cover and steam for three minutes until the vegetables are crisp. Combine the pineapple juice, cornflour and soy sauce and add to the wok together with the onions. Mix all the ingredients thoroughly until heated through. Serve immediately with the pre-prepared brown rice.

Dessert Recipes

Cherry Baked Apples

4 baking apples
½ tsp cinnamon
4 tbsp dried cherries or raisins
4 tbsp walnuts, chopped

Serves four

Preheat the oven to 375°F (190°C). Remove the apple cores without cutting the apples all the way through the outer end. Place the apples cored side up on a baking tray. Sprinkle the apples inside and outside with the cinnamon. Fill the apples with the cherries or raisins and the walnuts. Bake for 20 minutes until the apples are tender. Serve immediately.

Mixed Berry and Fruit Salad

200 g (7 oz) strawberries
juice of 2 limes
2 peaches
200 g (7 oz) raspberries
100 g (3½ oz) blackberries

Serves four

Cut the strawberries in half and pour over the lime juice. Stir carefully and marinate for half an hour. Stone and dice the peaches and mix with the raspberries and blackberries. Add the strawberries to the mix and serve.

How to Prepare and Eat Your Food

As well as eating the correct foods, the Healing Code places emphasis on eating the right way. The following ten-step approach to proper food preparation and consumption will ensure that you get the maximum benefit from the food that you eat:

1. Variety is encouraged as it ensures that you do not consume too much of the same ingredients, which could cause an internal imbalance.

2. There should be a strong preference for fresh ingredients. Fresh organic vegetables are strongly favoured over frozen vegetables, which according to Chinese medicine are considered to be starved of essential food energy.

3. Always make sure you wash fruit and vegetables thoroughly as they may have been exposed to chemical pesticides.

4. Ingredients should generally be shredded, diced or thinly sliced as this makes them much easier to digest.

5. The main method of cooking is stir-frying as foods cooked quickly in this manner are more likely to retain their nutrients. Steaming is also recommended for the same reason. Over-cooking and microwaving are generally discouraged as these methods damage the quality of the food's energy.

6. Foods are generally served at room temperature or warmer, and you are discouraged from eating food direct from the fridge. These cold foods have to be heated internally when consumed and this impairs the digestive process.

7. Meals are followed with a cup of green tea, jasmine tea or warm water as these are considered an aid to digestion.

8. Overeating is discouraged as this puts a strain on digestion. It is usually recommended that you should eat to a point where you are 80% full. Always choose quality over quantity.

9. Breakfast is usually considered the most important meal of the day, and all food is generally consumed before 6 p.m. There is a famous phrase 'Eat breakfast like a king, lunch like a prince and dinner like a pauper.' What this means is that you should endeavour to eat your larger meals earlier in the day. This gives your body a chance to burn the calories that you just ate. More importantly, it means that when you are sleeping, your body can work on healing itself and is not endeavouring to digest food that has been eaten later in the evening.

10. Always relax and sit comfortably when eating. This aids in the digestion of your food.

The Healing Code Detox, in Chapter Five, gives you more advice about cooking and implementing the Healing Code Nutrition Plan into your daily life.

In Summary

- Food is the most powerful medication you will ever take, and you should give yourself the best every day. Good food choices are the key to healthy nutrition. If your diet has contained lots of poor food choices, such as fast food and processed food, it is much easier to make a complete change than to slowly wean yourself off. This approach also delivers benefits much more quickly.

- Be aware of good and bad cholesterol and aim for a combination of fruit and vegetables and foods that are high in whole grains but low in saturated fats, trans fats, refined carbohydrates, dairy and salt.

- Supplements should never replace healthy nutrition, but there are clear health benefits to taking certain vitamin and mineral supplements regularly. Follow the supplement suggestions given on page 152, but aim to get your main source of vitamins from proper eating habits.

- When eating out, phone ahead and make sure that the restaurant will cater for your dietary requirements. More and more people are becoming health conscious, and restaurants are consequently generally very accommodating to healthy-food requests.

- Eating should be for pleasure. Use the suggestions in the Healing Code Menu to inspire enjoyable but healthy eating habits. Check out www.healing-code.com for other menu suggestions, and why not also create some of your own using the Healing Code principles?

The Healing Code Nutrition Plan identifies which food elements are optimal to encourage a surge in your health recovery. But what can we do about past indiscretions? What other environmental and lifestyle elements do we need to remove to further enhance the strength of your recovery? Next we need to look at cleaning out these toxic elements with the Healing Code Detox.

CHAPTER FIVE

Step Four: The Healing Code Detox

A wonderful fact about our body is that it naturally fights to heal itself. When we remove the elements that compromise this self-healing process, your body is supercharged to win the battle for health recovery. The Healing Code Detox addresses the particular behaviours and substances that are to be avoided or eliminated in order for you to boost your recovery powers. As well as identifying which elements compromise the healing process, the detox armours you with an arsenal of powerful and proven techniques that will help you conquer unhelpful addictions, cravings and behaviours.

Our modern lifestyle contains many hidden dangers, such as chemical additives and preservatives that can have adverse physical and mental effects. This chapter highlights potentially harmful substances in our food and environment and provides sensible advice on how to adjust our lifestyle when facing life-challenging illness.

How do we develop our preferences? When do our preferences become needs? Why do our needs become addictions? Problems are encountered when our intake is excessive or congested in certain areas. Congestion involves both reduced elimination function and an overconsumption of certain foods or substances. The most common enemies in these categories are caffeine, alcohol, nicotine, refined sugar and dairy products.

This aspect of the Healing Code – the fourth step – works on the following principles:

1. A primary cause of illness is the accumulation of unnecessary waste, resulting in poison retention and subsequently disease.

2. Your body is designed to support optimal function and gives signals when these toxins are introduced to your body.

3. Given the proper environment, your body has the power to heal itself and return to its normal healthy state.

The pattern of disease over the last 100 years has changed dramatically. In the Western world diseases such as measles, polio and tuberculosis no longer carry the same threat due to improved hygiene, better standards of living and advances in medicine. However, there has been a considerable increase in incidences of illnesses such as heart disease, diabetes, cancer and MS. Coincidently, this has paralleled man's increased exposure to toxins of the modern age.

The level of toxic chemicals found in our environment has never been higher in human history. The fact is that we have all been contaminated by toxic chemicals. We were never designed to encounter such a heavy onslaught, and as a result of our inability to break down these chemicals, they build up and play havoc with our bodies' systems. The consequence of this toxic poisoning has been the escalating volume of diseases such as asthma, heart disease, diabetes and cancer.

While we never set out to expose ourselves to chemical toxins, the simple act of living puts us in direct contact with harmful materials without us even realising it. When we eat foods exposed to pesticides, additives and pollutants, we are allowing these substances into our body. Our skin is exposed to chemicals in cosmetics and cosmetic procedures, detergents and toiletries. The air that we breathe is contaminated by car fumes, industrial waste and environmental pollutants.

It is very difficult to estimate the number of people who are suffering from chemical-related illnesses that have been triggered by toxic exposure. Because we all have a different genetic make-up and live in different environments, it is problematic for scientists to expose direct links between illnesses and toxic chemicals. Nevertheless, the increased incidence of modern illnesses and the paralleled increase in exposure to toxic chemicals can leave no doubt that toxin avoidance and elimination must be an important component of the Healing Code.

The good news is that the Healing Code Nutrition Plan is also the optimum dietary approach to combating the toxins we encounter in our food and drink. The Healing Code Nutrition Plan boosts our body's natural ability to eliminate toxins, soaking up the more constant toxins so that they can be expelled from our bodies. The Healing Code Detox will therefore first of all focus on ways to approach implementing the Nutrition Plan.

Conquering Food Cravings – the Revulsion Technique

In 1998 I changed my eating habits completely overnight. Foods that had been a central and regular part of my diet have never been eaten again from that day hence. For some people, such a radical change in their diet presents some challenges. Indeed, I had my own challenges. For as long as I could remember I had eaten enormous amounts of cheese, and for me, it was always the first food I would turn to as a snack. However, I used a number of methods to ensure a relatively easy and rapid transition to alternative healthier options. I soon saw the benefits of giving up cheese, and shortly after these initial challenges were overcome, the advantages of being dairy-free were so obvious that it was very easy to remain eating more healthily. Perhaps the most powerful technique I used to conquer my cravings involves the clever use of mental revulsion . . .

You might forget this, but many foods that become addictive are often not pleasant to taste when you first encounter them. Just as the first time anyone smokes is a time of nausea, the first time we encounter harmful foods our body usually rejects the taste. However, because of our own persistence and the mental conditioning of advertisements promoting these harmful foods, we manage to train our bodies to accept these poisons.

The revulsion technique is all about relearning what our bodies already knew in the first place – that these foods do us no good at all.

Imagine a dead rat lying at the side of the road. Its belly has been split open, and its guts have spilled out. Hundreds of maggots are feeding on the juicy find. My guess is that the clearer you get this image, the less likely you are to want to bite into a hamburger or anything else for that matter.

The revulsion technique is a powerful way of combating the mind games played by TV advertisers. Eating greasy, salty, sugary, chemical-loaded food is not natural. They associate eating their trash products with enjoyment and fun. They tell us that we deserve it. Have you ever noticed how often advertisers use comedians for their voiceovers? Subconsciously, many of us are used to laughter and enjoyment when we hear the voice of the comedian. At a subconscious level we often transfer this sense of joy and happiness to the product. As all this is happening at a subconscious level, we are often unaware of the implications. Despite the fact that we already know that these foods cause illness and a host of medical conditions, we still associate sugar, salt and greasy, fatty foods with pleasure and fool ourselves that we deserve it.

Our thinking becomes distorted. We become obsessed with the search for pleasure and forget the many harmful effects. Before long it is the junk-food manufacturers that are in control of our lives. As we dance to their tune like puppets on a string, we develop a host of warning signs that we overlook – gas, obesity, bloating, indigestion, skin problems and illness. But we continue to fool ourselves that it has been *our* choice.

The closer we are to experiencing pleasure, the more we become obsessed with it. We focus exclusively on the pleasure and decide that we want it again. We remember all about the enjoyment and forget about all the negative effects. When we want this pleasure, in our minds we will focus on the best part of the experience. As we replay the pleasure experience in our minds, the sense of anticipation increases. A drug addict focuses on the pleasure of feeding his craving whilst ignoring the detrimental effect on health, the loss of money, the pain of withdrawal and the harmful effects on friends and family. If they could look at the complete picture, they would not contemplate using drugs at all. Similarly with junk foods, if we forced ourselves to look at the entire picture, we would never eat the wretched stuff.

Do you really want to eat food that is going to prevent you from recovering your health? Of course the answer is no. But we usually try to combat compulsive eating just in the moments before eating. This is the least effective time to fight the compulsion. You must defeat the compulsion during normal times, when you are walking, sitting watching TV or driving. You need to ask yourself at these times, what do you really want? Do you really want to be someone who eats sugar and has to deal with all the associated strains on your health? You need to go over all the reasons for avoiding sugar and other harmful foods that you found addictive again and again until it enters your subconscious. When you do this often enough, the next time you encounter sugar, biscuits, cakes or chocolate you will be repelled without even thinking about it.

The Revulsion Effect

The interesting thing about the revulsion effect is that it can be created and amplified to the point of nausea at will. You can try it now. The first time you may have to focus intently on a dead rat or a hair in your soup, but with just a little practice you can create the revulsion effect at will.

The revulsion effect is a powerful tool to help you stop eating harmful foods that you may have eaten habitually during your life. It shuts off the pleasure tape and creates the opportunity for you to refocus on what you really want. It will allow you to jump out of the obsession cycle and give you the opportunity to look at the importance of your health-recovery goal.

You can use the revulsion technique to stop eating harmful foods. Simply cultivate the feeling of revulsion by focusing on something that makes you feel nauseous and say to yourself, 'I don't feel like having any of this food.' Leave the kitchen, or shop, and get moving. There is no harsh battle of will, no fighting any obsession, just one moment of feeling nausea and off you go. Each time you conquer a harmful food craving you will feel stronger and happier in the knowledge that you are moving forwards towards better health.

Creating the revulsion effect is simple. With just a little practice, you will be able to create the feeling quickly and easily. Practise using it. Open the refrigerator door, create revulsion, then do something else. Use it several times a day for two or three days and it will soon become a hugely powerful tool that will put you in control of your food choices. You should use revulsion:

- When you are not hungry and you are thinking about food.
- When you are overeating.
- While visualising foods you are going to quit.

Revulsion Exercise

Step One

Consider an unhealthy food that you have experienced cravings for. Let's use chocolate cake as an example. Now close your eyes and see the cake in front of you. Allow the feelings to come to you as if you were just about to taste the food.

Step Two

Now imagine a food that you find disgusting. Something that makes you feel completely nauseous. With eyes still closed, imagine mixing this food liberally in with the food that you had the craving for. So perhaps the chocolate cake becomes a chocolate and sardine cake (with heads still attached).

Step Three

Now visualise hundreds of live maggots crawling all over the cake. Notice that someone has already tried to start eating the dish. You know that someone has been there because you can see some vomit at the side of the plate where they weren't able to keep the food down.

Step Four

See yourself biting into the cake mixture and feel the gut-wrenching feeling of disgust as you gag on the food.

Feel like chocolate cake now? Practise this again and again and notice how your feelings towards unhealthy foods quickly begin to change.

The Healing Code Kitchen Clear-out

As a first step to adopting the Healing Code Nutrition Plan, it is recommended that you remove all unhealthy foods from your kitchen. If all members of the household want to protect themselves from illness and wish to adopt the Healing Code Nutrition Plan, then you can proceed directly with a full kitchen clear-out. If, however, you are the only member of the household implementing the plan, then you must create cupboard, fridge and kitchen space that is dedicated to the foods that you will eat as part of your health recovery.

In general, clear out all processed food and anything containing MSG, artificial sweeteners, preservatives, flavourings and colourings. There is a more detailed list of which foods are to be avoided and which are to be included in your diet and why on page 122, but the following will be a quick checklist when doing your kitchen clear-out. So, to get you on your way, clear out the following foods from your kitchen:

Fridge-freezer

Replace	With
Alcohol (beer, white wine, etc.)	Red wine
Butter	Organic extra-virgin olive oil
Cheese	Very low-fat cheese (less than 1% fat)
Chicken nuggets	Organic free-range chicken
Chips	Organic sweet potato
Eggs	Organic free-range eggs (max. four eggs per week)
Ice cream	Frozen homemade ice-pops made from 100% fruit juice
Margarine containing hydrogenated oil or trans fats	Organic extra-virgin olive oil
Mayonnaise	Fat-free mayonnaise, soy sauce or balsamic vinegar
Milk (full fat and semi-skimmed)	Skimmed milk, soya or rice milk
Pâté	Hummus
Processed meat and fish	Organic free-range chicken, turkey and fish
Red meat and pork	Organic free-range chicken, turkey and fish
Soft drinks	Fresh fruit juice – squeezed/juiced at home
Yoghurt	Low-fat organic yoghurt

Cupboards

Replace	With
Biscuits	Fresh fruit
Cakes	Fresh fruit
Canned food	Fresh fruit and vegetables

Chocolate	Dried fruit (without additives)
Coffee	Green or jasmine tea
Commercial breakfast cereals	Oatmeal and unsweetened, high-fibre, low-salt cereal
Crisps	Unsalted nuts
Jam and marmalade	Homemade puréed fruit
Popcorn	Unsalted nuts
Salt	Black pepper, garlic, dried herbs, spices, etc.
Salted nuts	Unsalted nuts
Stock cubes	Organic low-sodium stock cubes
Sugar	Organic honey
Sweets	Dried fruit (without additives)
Tea	Green or jasmine tea
Tinned and instant soup	Homemade soup made from organic vegetables
Tomato sauce	Freshly chopped tomatoes
White bread and rolls	Wholemeal bread
White flour	Wholegrain flour – spelt, kamut or wholewheat
White rice	Brown, basmati or wild rice

Cooking Utensils and Storage

Now that you have removed some of the more harmful foods, it makes good sense to continue your clear-out by removing items used in food preparation that can lead to contamination.

Avoid all plastic-based packaging such as cling film and plastic wrap. These contain carcinogenic substances, which can easily get transferred to the food they are used to wrap. The toxins in plastic wrap also have hormone-mimicking properties, which have been linked to reproductive cancers. Where possible, wrap items such as fruit, vegetables and fish in brown paper.

Cooking vessels and eating utensils should be made of glass, wood, porcelain and earthenware where possible. Non-stick cooking vessels can emit toxins from the synthetic lining. Aluminium pots and pans also increase toxic discharge. Stainless steel is fine for knives and forks.

Recommended Cooking Methods

The best methods of cooking are stir-frying and steaming. These methods are beneficial as they ensure the retention of vital nutrients and vitamins.

Stir-frying

Stir-frying is an easy and quick way to cook pieces of white meat, fish and vegetables over a high heat, with a minimum amount of extra-virgin olive oil. Sometimes a sauce or liquid can be added at the end of the cooking process, allowing the ingredients to be steamed briefly. With stir-frying, the food is constantly moved around in the pan or wok to allow an equal distribution of heat. Stir-frying is originally an oriental cooking technique and has become increasingly popular throughout the world.

Because stir-frying cooks food very quickly, there is a minimum amount of vitamin loss from vegetables during the process. The colour and texture of the food are also preserved. Typical stir-fry dishes contain just a small amount of meat or fish with relatively large quantities of vegetables, which is in line with the Healing Code Nutrition Plan guidelines.

Stir-frying in the Orient is traditionally done in a wok. Because of its round bottom, the wok allows the ingredients to fall to the bottom of the pan, where the heat is the most intense. The classic round-bottomed wok is designed for cooking over a flame, but flat-bottomed versions are available for use on electric hobs.

Careful preparation of ingredients is an important part of a successful stir-fry. Vegetables should be cut into small pieces to allow fast and even cooking. Cutting into smaller pieces also aids in the digestion process. Longer vegetables such as carrots are usually cut into strips or thinly sliced, round vegetables are cut into pieces, and broccoli and cauliflower are broken into small florets. It is usually the case that vegetables are cut at an angle to give them more surface area so that they cook more quickly. Fish and poultry are cut either into thin strips or wafer-thin slices, again so that it facilitates fast cooking. The protein elements – poultry, fish or tofu – are often marinated for a few hours to tenderise and to add flavour. It is important that all the ingredients are ready before the cooking process begins, including measuring out sauces and seasonings. As stir-fry cooking is so fast, there is no time for preparation between cooking steps.

When all of the ingredients are ready, the cooking process can begin. Start by heating the wok and then drizzle extra-virgin olive oil around the edge. The oil is quickly heated and coats the inside and bottom of the hot wok. When it is very hot, you can begin adding the first ingredients. The first ingredients added will usually be the flavouring ones such as ginger or garlic. These ingredients will flavour the oil very quickly. Then the poultry, fish or thicker vegetables are added (as they generally need to be cooked for longer). The other ingredients follow, with those that need the least cooking being added last. Throughout the cooking process the ingredients are stirred and tossed with a wooden spatula or by shaking the wok. The addition of a sauce is usually the last step of the cooking process. Once this thickens, the dish is ready to be served.

Steaming

The second Healing Code cooking method also originated in the Orient. Steaming has become increasingly popular in recent years, but it is in fact one of the oldest of all cooking methods. It is thought that steaming may even pre-date the discovery of fire, as it is believed that early man may have used the stones of hot springs to cook food.

Steaming simply involves cooking food in steam. In the West this generally means using a metal perforated basket placed over a saucepan. In the East food is generally steamed in bamboo steamers over a wok.

Steaming is considered a light and very healthy cooking method because no fat or oil at all is added. Mineral and vitamin loss are kept to an absolute minimum, so that all valuable nutrients are preserved. Similarly to stir-frying, the colours, flavours and textures of delicate ingredients are also retained. During the cooking process the food has no contact with the water. Steaming ensures that poultry and fish remain succulent.

There are many steamers available: special electrical steaming appliances, tiered pans with several steaming baskets, traditional bamboo steamers and petal steamers, which open up to fit most saucepans and fold away for easy storage.

When using steaming as a cooking method, use the following approach:

- Place the steamer over a saucepan of boiling water and fit the lid tightly to prevent the steam escaping. When the steam has built up, add the ingredients to the basket.
- Ensure that the steamer basket isn't touching the water, or the food will be boiled rather than steamed.
- Line the steamer with a muslin cloth to stop delicate food breaking up.
- Make sure the pan never boils dry. If necessary, keep a separate pot of boiling water close to hand in case you need to replenish the water in the saucepan.
- Remember, steaming doesn't add flavour so if necessary the food should be marinated, seasoned after cooking or served with a sauce.
- Remove vegetables from the steamer and serve as soon as the cooking time is over. Food that remains in the steamer continues to cook even if the heat is turned off, so vegetables can begin to discolour.

Other cooking methods are less healthy than stir-frying and steaming. For obvious reasons, you should avoid any method that requires you to use excessive amounts of oil or fat. Also avoid overcooking as this particularly robs your food of vital minerals and vitamins, the nutrients that are vital to a healthy recovery.

Cooking Methods to Avoid
Microwaving

Avoid microwave cooking as it robs your food, and hence your body, of vital nutrients. There is the possibility that microwaves may cause actual chemical changes in the food because of the intensity of the electromagnetic waves involved in the cooking process. They add potentially harmful toxins to your body as they absorb toxins from food packaging. There is also the danger of exposure to harmful electromagnetic radiation. If you have a microwave, stop using it or, better still, remove it from your kitchen completely.

Barbequing

Avoid eating barbequed food. The high temperatures involved in barbequing can frequently cause biochemical mutations in the food, particularly when charring has occurred. This has been linked to birth defects and cancer. A German study revealed that women who frequently partake of barbequed foods have twice the risk of developing breast cancer as women who never eat barbequed foods. Furthermore, the smoke produced from barbequing can contain benzopyrene – a dangerous carcinogen. A carcinogen is a substance or agent that may produce or incite cancer.

General Food Guidelines
Go Organic

The amount of pesticides used in crop production is staggering. Residues of these pesticides are in our foods and have been associated with many illnesses. Therefore an important step in reducing our exposure to pesticides is to eat organic foods wherever possible.

By going organic, you will help eliminate pesticide residues from your body. Studies have also shown that organic produce contains higher levels of vitamins and minerals.

Organic foods are now easy to find and they support your health recovery. With the increased demand for organic foods, prices are now more reasonable than ever before.

Washing Fruit and Vegetables

Wash all fruit and vegetables in filtered water to remove pesticide residues. This is particularly important for non-organic fruit and vegetables. Chemical pesticides are sprayed on crops to combat insects, weeds and rodents so as you can imagine, these chemical residues are detrimental to your health. Where appropriate, use a scrubbing brush and remove the outer layer and skin.

The Healing Code Dental Detox

It's true that most dentists will tell you that amalgam fillings are harmless. But let's face it, what else are they going to say? The bulk of scientific research, on the other hand, shows a different reality. All forms of mercury are toxic. Elemental mercury, the type that dental amalgam is derived from, is totally bio-available – in other words, it is absorbed by our bodies. Mercury from amalgam fillings has been shown to be neurotoxic and capable of causing a variety of immune dysfunctions and auto-immune diseases.

When asked if there was any safe level of mercury, Dr Lars Friberg, a world-leading authority on mercury poisoning and the former chief adviser to the World Health Organization on mercury safety, said he believes that there is 'no safe level of mercury, and no one has actually shown that there is a safe level. I would say mercury is a very toxic substance.'

Most people now know that the dental fillings in their mouths are made up mostly of the deadly substance. Amalgam fillings are 50% mercury and about 35% silver; the remaining 15% is a mixture of tin, zinc and copper. These fillings have been in use for about a hundred and eighty years, originating in England and spreading to Europe and America. At the time they were used by dentists because they provided a cheap and reasonably effective alternative to any other filling technique. It is generally accepted by the dentistry community that if amalgam was to require legal approval for use now, it would not be granted, because of the serious questions that remain about its safety.

What Dentists Are Taught About Amalgam

Dentists themselves are given very specific training in how to handle dental amalgam safely:

- They must not touch amalgam with their bare hands, as the mercury can enter the body through the skin.
- They must use thorough ventilation, as the mercury vapour produced from amalgam is easily absorbed into the body by inhalation.
- The amalgam taken out of teeth must be stored under photographic fixer in a sealed glass container. The high sulphur content of the solution helps to prevent release of mercury vapour into the atmosphere.
- It is illegal to dispose of waste amalgam into the sewerage system, as it will pollute the environment.
- Specialists in this field must dispose of waste amalgam as toxic waste.

Can you believe therefore that the only safe and legal place to keep this toxic waste is in the mouth of a living person? It just doesn't make any sense!

Prominent mercury researcher Dr Boyd Haley from the University of Kentucky points out, 'We can't go inside a living human being and look at their brain, so we have to work outside and do scientific experiments such as we've done. And to the best that we can determine with these experiments, mercury is a time bomb in the brain, waiting to have an effect. If it's not bothering someone when they're young, especially when they age it can turn into something quite disastrous.'

How Does Mercury Get Released From Your Teeth?

Mercury escapes from amalgam all the time. Each time you have a hot drink, chew or grind your teeth the level of mercury coming from the amalgam increases. So the majority of people with amalgam fillings will be living with a permanently elevated level of mercury vapour in their mouths.

In 1991 the World Health Organization recognised that dental amalgam constituted the greatest source of mercury to the general population and that there was no level of mercury vapour that was found to be harmless. In fact, autopsy studies have shown that the level of mercury in the brain is directly proportional to the number of amalgam fillings in the mouth.

How Can Mercury Affect Your Health?

Up to 80% of inhaled mercury vapour is absorbed through the lungs. According to a report in the prestigious medical journal the *Lancet*, a percentage of mercury vapour adheres to the lining of the nose and mouth and is transported directly into the brain. Mercury from amalgam easily crosses the blood-brain barrier and damages the whole of the central nervous system. Some mercury is also transported along the nerve fibres back to the brain. Mercury has been found all the way down the spinal cord. According to the report, this may result in symptoms similar to motor neurone disease and sensations of pain, itching and tingling throughout the body. Minute amounts of mercury in the brain will cause the same type of damage as is found in the brains of patients with Alzheimer's disease.

True allergy to amalgam is only one type of immune reaction. There is extensive scientific research discussing the damaging effects mercury has on the immune system. Mercury from amalgam may result in an increase in allergies, skin rashes and itching. If mercury has a detrimental effect on the immune system, this will create an environment in the body for other diseases to develop. When mercury binds to proteins, these proteins will appear to the cells of the immune system as foreign substances. They will then be attacked by the immune system and may lead to a cascade of events ending in possible auto-immune diseases.

Mercury is a cumulative poison. It remains in your body, and the level is topped up continuously. This form of poisoning is called micromercurialism. The earliest symptoms are subclinical neuro-logical – fatigue, headaches, forgetfulness, reduced short-term memory, poor concentration, shyness and timidity, confusion, rapid mood swings, unprovoked anger, depression and suicidal tendencies.

Mercury from amalgam fillings has also been shown in animal studies to cause a 50% reduction in kidney filtration after just two months in the mouth. This indicates a great reduction in the ability of the kidneys to eliminate toxic waste from your body. Mercury therefore compromises your body's natural ability to detoxify and heal itself.

What Can You Do?

After reading this, it is tempting for people to be concerned enough to rush to their dentist and demand that all of their amalgams be replaced. But make sure only to go to a dentist who specialises in replacing amalgam fillings. Unless you take the appropriate precautions, you could expose yourself even more to high levels of mercury. There is a proper approach to the safe removal of amalgam, which has been designed to maximise the benefit of this type of treatment for the patient. Removing amalgam fillings will stop the greatest source of mercury into your body, but mercury will still be stored in your body and takes time to come out.

For future visits to your dentist, never allow amalgam to be placed in your mouth ever again. There are alternatives, and replacement with natural-looking bonded materials is a common holistic dentistry treatment, as well as a common cosmetic dentistry treatment. If your dentist still believes that the alternatives are not as good as amalgam, perhaps you could suggest he or she reads the published literature demonstrating that amalgam is in fact one of the worst mechanical restorative materials. Alternatively, you can change dentists – you do have the right to choose.

Even if you do not have your amalgams removed, there are some dietary supplements that have been shown to be helpful either to remove mercury from the body or to start to repair some of the damage caused by mercury. A good mercury-free dentist should support the detoxification process. Research released in 1996 has shown that fresh coriander can successfully attach to mercury that has already reached the brain and remove it back across the blood-brain barrier (BBB). Two of the Healing Code Nutrition Plan's supplements also help remove mercury from your body: spirulina and selenium. Mercury will bind strongly to selenium, the trace element needed for a wide variety of enzyme functions. Latest research indicates a direct relationship between reduced blood selenium levels and an increase in the rate of cancer.

You can locate a mercury-free dentist in the UK or Ireland by contacting:

The British Society for Mercury-Free Dentistry
PO Box 42606
London SW5 OXA

Helpline: 020 8746 1177
www.mercuryfreedentistry.org.uk

The Healing Code Environmental Detox

The level of chemicals and pollutants that we are exposed to is at an all-time high. When we think of harmful chemicals, most of us will think of a smoggy, polluted urban area. Unfortunately, many of the harmful toxins are found in our very homes, and because of our regular proximity, they potentially do more harm than the smoke-belching factory.

Not only do we face these toxins in our food, but body creams, tanning lotions and many beauty products contain chemicals that potentially compromise our immune systems and are therefore a barrier to health recovery. Whilst it is practically impossible to avoid all harmful chemicals, it is possible to dramatically decrease your exposure by simply paying more attention to the products that you use in your household, garden and on your body. It will again involve a clear-out and making certain changes, but the benefits will be repaid with an even greater surge in your health recovery.

Make the following key changes:

- Remove tobacco smoke from your home. If any of your friends or family want to smoke, they are free to do so outside. As second-hand tobacco smoke contains over four thousand chemicals, many of which are carcinogenic, there is no place for this in your home. If you are the one producing these chemicals by smoking, follow the Healing Code Nicotine Detox on page 197.
- Clear out all your domestic-cleaning products, as they generally contain a large quantity of toxic chemicals. Consider healthier alternatives such as vinegar and water for cleaning windows, lemon juice for cleaning dishes and bathroom areas, and baking soda and water for cleaning ovens. Undiluted white vinegar can be used as a household disinfectant. A number of environmentally safe cleaning products are readily available. The Ecover brand has a variety of products that safely provide for all your domestic-cleaning needs.
- Throw out all artificial air fresheners. Although some may smell pleasant, they do so by frequently emitting toxic odours that can cause cancer. These hazards contain such lethal substances as ethanol, formaldehyde, phenol and xylene. As an alternative, use proper ventilation together with natural essential oils on flower-based pot-pourri.
- When using scented candles, make sure that they are made from plant or beeswax and that they contain only pure essential oils and not synthetic fragrances.
- Remember to use your kitchen extractor fan and make sure that it is vented outside.
- Avoid exposure to all products that contain methylene chloride and benzene. Methylene chloride is found in paint strippers and aerosol spray paint and has been found to cause cancer in animals. Benzene, found in paint, has been found to cause cancer in humans.
- If you are redecorating your living room, try to use natural furnishings that have not been treated by chemicals. Consider natural wood flooring as an alternative to carpet, which usually contains volatile organic compounds. If you already have a

carpet and wish to have it cleaned, have it steam-cleaned without the use of toxic chemicals.

The Healing Code Skincare Detox

We all want to look our best, but most of us fail to realise that many of the body and skincare products that we use are overloaded with toxic chemicals. Perfumes, make-up, deodorants and shampoos often contain toxins that are harmful to our bodies. A significant benefit of detoxification is that you are far less inclined to even need many of these personal-care products to enhance your appearance. Detoxification improves your skin and appearance naturally.

The Healing Code Skincare Detox therefore suggests the following changes:

- When using body creams and beauty products, choose natural, environmentally friendly products. Because of the increased awareness of the dangers of chemicals in cosmetic products, the market has responded with many manufacturers providing a safe and extensive range of skincare products. The small additional cost will yield a significant health dividend.
- Cut down or eliminate the use of perfumes and colognes. These are frequently made from petrochemicals and other synthetic toxic materials, which can compromise your immune system. Instead, pick natural essential oils from plant sources to create hydrosols, which can be sprayed or used from dropper bottles.
- Studies have shown that as many as 20% of non-Hodgkin's lymphoma cases are related to the use of artificial hair colouring. There is an increased risk of illnesses such as multiple myeloma, leukaemia and Hodgkin's disease if you frequently use hair dyes over a long period of time. There are now a variety of non-toxic, plant-based and biodegradable hair colourants available. So if you do colour your hair, endeavour to use these natural products at all times.
- Use flouride-free toothpaste. There is a debate about the safety of

fluoride with suggestions that it is a contributor to increased cancer risk as well as a variety of other diseases. You don't have to wait to see who wins the debate. It is just common sense to avoid excessive fluoride if you are recovering your health.

- Avoid using commercial deodorants and antiperspirants. These products frequently contain harmful ingredients such as aluminium, which has been associated with Alzheimer's disease, triclosan, which has been linked to liver damage, and colourings, which are suspected carcinogens.
- Bring plants into your home as they combat air pollution. Do remember to remove plants from your bedroom at night-time, when plants generally absorb oxygen and release carbon dioxide.
- In order to keep your exposure to the chemical content of clothing to a minimum, try to wear clothes made of natural fibres. When washing your clothes, again use an environmentally safe washing powder such as Ecover. If you need to get your clothes dry-cleaned, always make sure to air these items before putting them back in your wardrobe.

The Healing Code Nicotine Detox

If you smoke, becoming a non-smoker is perhaps the single most important thing you can do to bring you towards health recovery – no matter what your illness is. Smoking causes so much direct and indirect damage to your body that kicking this habit must be given immediate priority. Why would you start eating pure and healthy food and continue to inhale literally thousands of toxic chemicals into your lungs?

You may be surprised how soon you start to see benefits when you have stopped smoking.

Some Facts About Quitting
Within 20 minutes of smoking that last cigarette, your body begins a series of changes that continue for years.

Twenty minutes after quitting
Your heart rate and blood pressure drop to a level close to that before your last cigarette.
The temperature of your hands and feet increases, returning to normal.

Twelve hours after quitting
The carbon monoxide level in your blood drops to normal.
The oxygen level in your blood increases to normal.

Twenty-four hours after quitting
Your heart-attack risk begins to drop.

Forty-eight hours after quitting
Your nerve endings start regrowing.
Your ability to smell and taste is enhanced.

Two weeks to three months after quitting
Your lung function improves by up to 30%.
Your circulation improves.
Walking becomes easier.

One to nine months after quitting
Cilia regrow in lungs, increasing your ability to handle mucus, cleaning the lungs and lowering your risk of lung infections. Your lungs start to function better.
Your body's overall energy increases.

One year after quitting
Your added risk of coronary heart disease is half that of a smoker.

Five years after quitting
Your stroke risk is reduced to that of someone who has never smoked.

How to Quit Smoking

The Healing Code offers some powerful techniques that you can use to remove nicotine from your life for good. If you are recovering from illness, that easily provides all the motivation you need to conquer smoking. The chances are that smoking has contributed in some shape or form to the health predicament you are in. Use all of these techniques regularly and you will soon see the health rewards of being a non-smoker.

In preparation for quitting, do the following:

- The first few days, drink *lots* of water and fluids to help flush out the nicotine and other poisons from your body.
- Tell friends and family members that you are quitting and ask for their support and encouragement. Once you ask for support you'll be surprised how much it can help and how much motivation it provides for you to succeed.
- Ask friends and family members not to smoke in your presence. Don't be afraid to ask. This is more important than you may realise.
- On your quit day, hide all ashtrays and destroy all your cigarettes, preferably with water.
- If there are any places in particular where you used to smoke, change the layout of those places. Move the seats, or change the location of the phone. Our brains create a lot of associations around smoking and these can be broken simply by making some small changes.

Techniques for Giving Up Smoking

Technique One

Deep breathing is perhaps the most powerful technique for anyone who is stopping smoking. If you feel any cravings for a cigarette, do the following three times. People often mistakenly believe that they relax when smoking because of nicotine. Although it is true that people relax when they smoke, it is simply because this is the only time when they breathe deeply.

1. Inhale your deepest breath and fill your lungs. Then, very gently, exhale. Purse your lips so that the air comes out very slowly.
2. As you exhale, close your eyes and let your chin gradually sink on to your chest. Visualise all the tension leaving your body, slowly draining out of your fingers and toes, just flowing out.

When you practise this, you'll be able to use it for *any* future stressful situation you find yourself in. It will be your greatest weapon during any cravings. The best thing is that each and every time you succeed with the technique its power increases.

Technique Two

Get a sheet of paper and write down the six main reasons from the following list why you don't like smoking, why it's bad and you have stopped:

1. Cigarette smoking makes smokers age prematurely. A smoker in her forties may have as many wrinkles as a non-smoker in her sixties.
2. Smoking increases the risk of impotence by around 50% for men in their thirties and forties.
3. Female smokers have more trouble getting pregnant than non-smokers and also have a higher rate of miscarriage during pregnancy.
4. Smoking makes your breath, hair and clothes stink.
5. Teeth and fingers get stained brown with nicotine.
6. A typical pack-a-day smoker spends over £150 a month and £1,825 a year.
7. One in five people die from illnesses directly linked to smoking.
8. If you smoke regularly for a long time, you may get a disease called peripheral vascular disease. This disease causes narrowing of the blood vessels, which restricts blood flow to the hands and feet, leading to gangrene and the amputation of limbs.
9. Smoking messes up your body chemistry. It decreases the levels of vitamin C in your blood, for example. Vitamin C, among other things, protects you against carcinogens, boosts immunity and

helps prevent heart disease. And smoking increases cholesterol. It's estimated that every cigarette you smoke raises your total cholesterol by about half a point.

10. Smokers have a higher frequency of severe depression, anxiety disorders and other psychological problems.

11. If you smoke, you have an increased risk of gum disease, muscle injury, angina, neck pain, back pain, abnormal eye movements, circulatory disease, fungal eye infection, ulcers, osteoporosis, cataracts, Crohn's disease, pneumonia, depression, psoriasis, type-two diabetes, skin wrinkling, hearing loss, flu, rheumatoid arthritis and tendon and ligament injuries – among other conditions.

12. Smoking causes cancer. The links between cigarettes and cancer of the oral cavity, oesophagus, lungs, kidneys, pancreas, stomach, cervix and bladder are indisputable.

Next, on the other side of the sheet, write down all the reasons why you'll feel great when you've succeeded in stopping. You'll feel healthier, your sense of taste and smell will be enhanced, your hair and clothes will smell fresher and so on. When you have finished, fold this sheet of paper and carry it where you used to carry your cigarettes.

Technique Three

Next, we are going to use the revulsion technique to reprogramme your mind to feel disgusted by cigarettes. Recall four times when you thought to yourself, 'I've got to quit smoking', or when you felt disgusted about smoking. Maybe you remember getting a diagnosis from your doctor because of your smoking and he told you that 'You've got to quit', or somebody you know was badly affected by smoking. Take a moment now to come up with four separate occasions when you felt that you had to quit or were disgusted by smoking.

Close your eyes and remember each of those times as though they are happening right now. Jump from each memory to the other and keep going through each until you can make them as vivid as possible.

See what you saw, hear what you heard and feel how you felt. Take some time now and go through those memories again and again. Rapidly overlap each memory with the next until you feel totally and utterly disgusted by cigarettes.

Technique Four

Have you ever heard of an adult who continues to carry a blanket or 'blankie' around that they had as a baby? The human mind is very sensitive to associations, and in this case the person as an infant has associated comfort and safety with the blanket. Subconsciously they have tricked themselves into believing that this sense of comfort has emanated from the blanket itself.

In a similar way, people become accustomed to cigarettes in certain situations. If you smoked whilst taking a break and chatting to work colleagues, subconsciously you fool yourself into thinking that the relaxation of taking a break and the enjoyment of talking to friends is due to the cigarette. This of course is just as delusional as the blankie being a source of safety. So, now that you have quit smoking, continue to give yourself relaxation times but do something different. Go for a walk or chat with a friend.

Technique Five

Several times a day quietly repeat to yourself the affirmation 'I am a non-smoker.' Many quitters see themselves as smokers who are just not smoking for the moment. Silently repeating the affirmation 'I am a non-smoker' will help you change your view of yourself, and even if it may seem silly to you, this is actually useful. Use it!

Technique Six

You used to use cigarettes to signal to your body to release happy chemicals, so next we are going to programme some powerfully positive feelings into your future.

Sit comfortably and recall a time when you felt very deep pleasure. Take a moment to remember it as vividly as possible. Remember the detail – see what you saw, hear what you heard and feel how good you felt.

Keep going through the memory. As soon as it finishes, go through it again and again, all the time squeezing your thumb and forefinger together. That's right: see what you saw, hear what you heard and feel how good you felt. Make the pictures big, bright and vivid, the sounds loud and crisp, and the feelings strong. Again, squeeze your thumb and forefinger together. This creates an associational link between the squeeze of your fingers and that great feeling.

OK, now stop and relax. If you have done this correctly, whenever you squeeze your thumb and finger together you should feel that good feeling again. Go ahead and do that now: squeeze thumb and finger and remember that good feeling. Keep practising this over and over.

Now you are going to programme good feelings to happen automatically whenever you are in a situation where you used to smoke.

Next I'd like you to squeeze your thumb and forefinger together, get that great feeling going and imagine being in a situation where you would have smoked but you are there feeling great without a cigarette. Take that good feeling into those situations without the need for a cigarette.

Imagine being in a situation where someone offers you a cigarette and you smile confidently say, 'No, thanks, I don't smoke!' And feel good about it!

Here is perhaps the most valuable of all points. In the second phase, which begins a few weeks after quitting, the urge to smoke will subside considerably. However, it's vital to understand that occasionally you may still get a desire for 'just one cigarette'. This will happen unexpectedly, during moments of stress, whether negative stress or positive (at a party or on holiday). If you are unprepared to resist, succumbing to that 'one cigarette' may lead you directly back to smoking. Remember the following secret: in these surprise attacks do the next thought-field therapy exercise, hold on for five minutes and the urge will pass.

Thought-Field Therapy – the Powerful Addiction Cure

If you are feeling addictive cravings for food, nicotine or anything at all, or are just feeling generally stressed and want to reduce that feeling immediately, you can once again use the powerful technique thought-field therapy. The following is very similar to the version we used to eliminate fears in Chapter Three. Turn to page 109 for a more detailed explanation of the origin and role of thought-field therapy. It is important to think about the craving or anxiety throughout this exercise.

1. Concentrate on the craving or thing that is causing you stress and rate it on a scale of one to ten, with one being a weak craving and ten being strong. Write down the rating so that you can see how much it has reduced at the end of the exercise.
2. Using two fingers of one hand, while still thinking of the craving, tap five times under the collarbone.
3. Tap five times under the eye on the bony part of the cheekbone.
4. Tap the collarbone again five times, whilst thinking of the craving.
5. Now, placing your other hand out in front of you, tap rapidly on the back of your hand between your ring finger and little finger. Still thinking of the craving and whilst continuing to tap rapidly:
   - Open and close your eyes.
   - Open your eyes and look down to the left.
   - Look down to the right.
   - Circle your eyes round 360 degrees clockwise.
   - Circle your eyes round 360 degrees anticlockwise.
   - Hum the first few lines of 'Happy Birthday' out loud.
   - Count aloud from one to five.
   - Hum a few lines of 'Happy Birthday' again.
6. Tap firmly under the collarbone five times.
7. Tap firmly under the eye five times.
8. Tap firmly under the collarbone five times.

Now check how much your craving has decreased. Rate the craving again on the one to ten scale. If the craving hasn't disappeared completely, simply go through the sequence again until it does. Most people will find that they can completely eliminate any craving with just one or two repetitions. Perform the exercise until the craving has disappeared.

If the craving comes back, repeat the process again as often as you like.

In Summary

- It's time to banish unhealthy habits. Use the Healing Code Kitchen Clear-out and the revulsion technique on page 179 to help implement your healthy nutrition plan.
- Use healthier cooking methods as well as cooking materials that do not expose you unnecessarily to toxic residues.
- In time consider your potential exposure to mercury poisoning, and certainly in the future avoid amalgam fillings.
- Smoking is one of the main causes of heart and lung disease, as well as a host of other conditions. Therefore avoid exposure to second-hand smoke.
- If you are the one who is smoking, now is the time to free yourself from this harmful habit. Use the techniques in this chapter to give up nicotine.
- Address other harmful chemical addictions by using the powerful addiction cure thought-field therapy.

Having addressed your exposure to harmful toxins, your body is supercharged to heal itself and return itself to a normal healthy state. Continuing to fuel your body with the foods of the Healing Code Nutrition Plan will support your recovery. But just as stagnant waters become unhealthy and harbour disease, our bodies – which are mostly water – also need to be kept moving. This leads us to the fifth and final element of the Healing Code – the most powerful exercise prescription for total health recovery – medical chi kung.

CHAPTER SIX

Step Five: The Healing Code Chi Kung Programme – the Ultimate Exercise Prescription

What Is Chi Kung?

The Chinese term 'chi kung' is made up of two words: 'chi', which is interpreted as 'life energy', and 'kung', meaning skill. Chi kung is therefore the ancient Chinese science where one learns awareness of this life energy and how to control its flow through posture, movement, respiratory technique and meditation. Chi kung teaches psychophysiological self-regulation: students can learn how to control bodily functions conventionally considered involuntary – blood pressure, respiratory rate, even the flow of blood and nutrients to internal organs – and hence restore a healthier balance.

Scientific studies in the West have proven that chi kung naturally improves the efficiency of respiratory delivery, as well as the activities of the nervous, hormone, digestive and immune systems. Studies have also shown that chi kung practice dramatically increases levels of the powerful antioxidant enzyme superoxide dismutase (SOD) in the bloodstream. This enhanced antioxidant activity scientifically verifies that chi kung retards the ageing process and helps to fight degenerative illnesses.

Chi kung is included in the Healing Code because it is simply the most powerful and cost-effective self-healing method in the world. Chi kung is easy to learn, and your only investment needed is time – about an hour each day. Over 120 million people practise chi kung in the world today, making it the world's most popular health exercise system.

Chinese medicine is based on an energetic model of medicine in contrast to Western medicine's biochemical model. Although these models are different, the health advice, medical concepts and theories about health and disease are often remarkably similar in both systems. In China, traditional Chinese medicine operates harmoniously side by side with Western medicine.

Chinese medicine knew about the circulation of blood within the body thousands of years before Western medicine 'discovered' it. Chinese medical surgery was pioneered in China some 1,500 years before surgeries were performed in the West.

According to Chinese medicine, when ill, a person's life energy flows excessively or weakly through the body compared to when in good health. When chi is properly cultivated or managed in the body through kung, a person remains in good mental, emotional and physical health.

Perhaps it is in the field of cancer that chi kung has shown the most dramatic results. Amongst the millions of cancer patients practising chi kung in the East, there are a vast number of successful cases of aided cancer recovery. Thousands of cases have been documented with case studies for every type of cancer. Patients have often not only recovered from cancer but have also had their overall health and vitality completely restored.

The Benefits of Exercise

Many claims have been made about the health benefits of physical exercise. The scientific evidence is now overwhelmingly strong in support of the advantages of exercise for health recovery. Physical activity affects both mind and body. The beneficial consequences of exercise include some obvious elements – reduction of blood pressure, lower pulse rate and less body fat. But new evidence is showing that physical exercise offers even more profound benefits. As well as helping muscles, the heart and lungs, physical exercise supports a more fundamental aspect of healthy recovery – the immune response. Moderate exercise can elicit increases in several immune-function measures, including the cell-eating activity of white blood cells, stimulating the immune system by raising interleukin levels, as well as increasing the number and activity of natural killer cells.

Physical exercise is, however, a two-edged sword. When exercise is intense and excessive, it can do harm. Extreme physical exercise is a powerful stressor and can actually impair immune function, lowering your body's defences against infection. Top athletes may be very fit, but it does not follow through that they are extremely healthy. Physical fitness and prowess have been the main goal of most Western exercise systems. In Eastern countries, however, the systems of exercise that developed were primarily focused on health and self-healing. Therefore it is common sense that if you want to harness the powerful healing effect of physical exercise, you should look to the Eastern systems of exercise that have a richer knowledge and a tradition which has evolved over thousands of years. It is for this reason that when I was diagnosed with MS I looked to Chinese medicine's exercise system chi kung.

I began studying Chinese medicine soon after I was diagnosed with MS. I was struck by the simple yet profound logic of this powerful medical system. Chinese medicine has developed through observation of human behaviour and health. Learned Chinese doctors noticed how patterns of lifestyle behaviours, food, emotions and the environment affected our bodies and our health. Whilst Western medicine floundered for an explanation for my condition, Chinese medicine gave a logical, multidimensional reason why MS developed within my body. It does the same for almost all illnesses and can work hand in hand with conventional medicine, as it does in China today. Indeed, Chinese medicine's ancient explanations for the lifestyle causes of cancer and heart disease have been verified as correct only in recent years after decades of Western medical research. If we look at something as simple as the common cold, Chinese medicine has long recognised that what your grandmother said was correct: you should wrap up warmly to avoid exposure to the cold. It might surprise you that it was only in 2005 that conventional medical science proved that being chilly can cause a cold to develop. A hundred and eighty volunteers at the University of Cardiff were subjected to 20 minutes with their feet immersed in ice-cold water, while the others sat with their feet in an empty bowl. During the next four or five days almost a third (29%) of the 'chilled' volunteers developed cold symptoms – compared to just 9% in the control group.

Whilst past research had dismissed any relationship between chilling and viral infection as having no scientific basis, new science has confirmed what Chinese doctors have known all along: the common cold, known in Chinese medicine as 'wind cold invading the body', is affected and often caused by the temperature of your body.

Chinese medicine has been around for some five thousand years and so there is an obvious wealth of documented knowledge about almost every disease and illness known to man. The newer diseases of the modern world such as AIDS and SARS have been vigorously studied by Chinese doctors, and powerful and effective treatment approaches continue to evolve.

On my first day at acupuncture school I learned of the four branches of Chinese medicine – acupuncture, herbal medicine, Chinese massage therapy and Chinese medicine's exercise system – medical chi kung. Chi kung is considered by many to be the oldest branch of Chinese medicine. Chi kung is also considered by many to be Chinese medicine's most powerful healing system.

It has been scientifically established that chi kung exercise offers compelling benefits to those recovering from life-challenging illnesses. These include improving heart and lung function, increasing blood supply to muscles and the ability to use oxygen, lowering heart rate and blood pressure, as well as increasing HDL cholesterol (the good cholesterol). There is a wealth of scientific evidence gathered in China and now in the West that chi kung can be used to treat a myriad of illnesses.

It is hard to overestimate the immense power of some chi kung exercises. Chi kung walking has been used for thousands of years to treat cancer in China. Modern scientific evidence is again just beginning to shed light on this powerful treatment approach, with some staggering statistics coming from research at some of the world's leading medical universities: as prevention, walking for one

hour a day cuts the risk of develop,
endometrial cancer by 30%, colon can
by 40%, stroke by 50% and diabetes by 5

In a large study of breast-cancer pati
Women's Hospital, which is affiliated to Har
cut their risk of fatality by walking at an avera
five hours a week. Bear in mind also that these s
to standard walking exercise. Chi kung walking has
over centuries specifically for disease prevention and   -y. Chi
kung walking therefore delivers results more impressiv- than these
already remarkable findings. Chi kung walking – explained later in
this chapter – incorporates powerful mind techniques together
with synchronised breathing methods.

Whilst in the West most exercise systems have their foundation
in improving sporting performance, chi kung is primarily aimed at
promoting health and has long-established methods of health
recovery purely through breathing, meditation and movement
exercises.

This chapter explains some of the key principles of chi kung.
This will enable you to establish a personalised system of exercise
that will boost the potency of the healing effect. Chi kung is a
powerful psychosomatic regime, which will aid in the prevention
and treatment of diseases.

The Healing Code Chi Kung Programme, which is the fifth step
in your health recovery, has been adopted for ease of use and works
on the three primary principles of chi kung energy correction –
moving stagnant energy, tonification and regulation. Particularly
helpful (and not available in most chi kung texts) will be the
mental focus of each exercise. The chapter includes the following:

- correct chi kung posture, breathing and mental focus
- building and absorbing energy
- removing stagnant energy – the key to chi kung cancer treatment
- digestion regulation – the Five Yang Organ Exercise
- The Five Yin Organ Exercise – strengthening lung, kidney, liver, heart and spleen

g the energy in your body – Kwan Gong Stroking Beard
ung walking exercises for cancer treatment.

When you are recovering from an illness, you might feel reluctant to do exercise. The fantastic thing about chi kung is that it is designed for the specific purpose of maintaining and regaining health. Therefore the chi kung exercises that you will perform will not strain your body, but rather will reinvigorate you and surge you towards a powerful state of well-being.

Starting Exercising

The time to start exercise is now. If you have not exercised before, you will still find chi kung very accommodating to your body. But as you are recovering your health, remember never to push yourself to exhaustion. We want your energy to build up, and training to exhaustion depletes your energy. This is one of the most common mistakes that people make when starting to do exercise and it defeats the purpose. The aim is to feel good before and after training and never to feel uncomfortable.

When you begin, you may wish only to exercise for five or ten minutes, depending on how good you feel. As time goes on, you will increase the duration of your training until you are able to exercise for between an hour and 90 minutes each day. But when you are just starting, go slowly. Give your body time to catch up with the eagerness your head has to recover your health.

Always seek your doctor's advice before exercising. Your training programme must also take into consideration days when you feel less inclined to train, whether it's due to tiredness or the effects of medical treatment. Listening to your body and also becoming aware of your emotional state is key to effective chi kung training. Often when you feel tired it may be due to emotional stresses. Chi kung training is very effective at relieving these stresses. However, you must listen to your body, and when you are genuinely tired, then you must take a break from training.

Chi Kung Frequently Asked Questions

What equipment do I need to practise chi kung?

No special equipment, uniform or grounds are required to practise chi kung, and it can be done at any time and in any place. All you need is a small amount of open space, some loose, comfortable clothing and some comfortable shoes.

Is chi kung easy to learn?

Yes! The chi kung movements are not physically hard on the body or strenuous, and while there are a few movements that the new student may find challenging at first, on the whole chi kung is very easy to learn. There is no age limit with chi kung – both young and old can practise and gain health benefits from it. Chi kung can even be performed while seated.

When is the best time to practise chi kung?

The best times to practise chi kung are first thing in the morning and last thing in the evening before retiring to bed. Practising in the morning will adjust your body and mind for the remainder of the day. When you practise before retiring at night, several hours after dinner, it will help you to wind down and lead you into a restful sleep. Remember that these are guidelines. If the afternoon is more convenient for you, then that's when you train. The important thing is that you do practise.

How often should I train?

You should aim to practise chi kung every day. When recovering your health, always allow your energy to build up and refrain from training to exhaustion. This could mean not performing the full training programme on all days.

What should I do if I experience pain or discomfort from a particular exercise?

Proper posture is very important to prevent discomfort. Many have a lifetime of poor posture leading to weak muscles, ligaments and tendons. Correcting your posture during exercise often results in the student experiencing shakiness, cramping or soreness in weak muscles and joints. Focus on correct posture and over a period of weeks gradually increase the time you spend in a static position. If standing posture causes you discomfort, it is perfectly acceptable to perform the exercises whilst seated.

For how long should I practise?

This will vary from individual to individual, but again the key point to remember is that when exercising for health recovery you should never train to exhaustion. Twenty minutes' practice in the morning, with half an hour chi kung walking during the day, concluding with twenty minutes' practice before retiring at night represents a solid chi kung training regime.

How long will it take me to experience chi, and what is it like?

That depends. Everyone has experienced it indirectly, such as the buzzing feeling of having your foot fall asleep when you've knelt for too long. Some learn quickly how to identify the sensation of chi in the exercises, while others may experience it only after many months or years of practice. Ultimately, it is best not to worry about it. Things happen in their own good time. Mental intention and deep relaxation will help you progress.

What can I expect to feel during practice?

What one really feels is the effect of energy movement in the body rather than feeling energy directly. The effect has been commonly described as a feeling of warmth or coolness, or a magnetic-like, itching or buzzing sensation.

What are the benefits of chi kung?

Chi kung provides the following key benefits: 1) better health, 2) sounder sleep, 3) increased strength, 4) clearer skin, 5) more efficient and active metabolism and 6) improved psychological outlook. In short, you will begin to feel great again.

Should I attend a chi kung class?

By all means attend a local chi kung class. The exercises might be different, but they should be based on the same principles. The important thing is that you find a good teacher who is able to explain in clear English all three aspects of chi kung exercise – physical movements, breathing technique and mental intention. From my experience, it is usually easy to find a teacher who can teach the first two aspects, but difficult to find a teacher who can or is willing to explain the mental aspect of the exercise system. Always bear in mind, however, that the mental aspect of chi kung training is the most important element and it is the key to successful practice. The Healing Code Chi Kung Programme is easy to learn, and provided you take the time to practise, you will have great success. The supporting DVD available from *www.healing-code.com* may also prove useful for learning to perform the exercises correctly.

Getting Started – the Basics of the Programme

This form of chi kung training was brought to the West by Dr Her Yue Wong and brought to me by my teacher in the US, Jerry Alan Johnson. These techniques have become very popular because they are both very simple to learn and very effective.

There are three stages in learning chi kung exercises. Stage one is where you are developing physical familiarity, where you learn, practise and perfect the physical movement of the exercise. Stage two is where you learn to coordinate correct breathing with the physical movements. Stage three is where you focus your mental intention on thoughts coordinated with these movements. It is this final stage that makes chi kung different from Western exercise systems. It is also within this stage that all the true power of chi kung exists. Only when you have perfected the physical movements and coordinated your breathing without needing any conscious effort can you focus full mental intention on the visualisations associated with the exercises. The exercises that I have chosen for this programme have been selected for their simplicity, as they allow you to get to stage three as quickly and effectively as possible. Before long you will have perfected the physical movements and breathing techniques and will be ready to unleash the potent healing power of chi kung.

Correct Chi Kung Posture

For the Healing Code Chi Kung Programme there are two recommended postures – sitting and standing. It is very important that you do not exhaust yourself when you are recovering from ill health. Therefore, if you do not wish to stand for 30 minutes, it is quite acceptable to sit for all or part of the programme.

Correct sitting posture includes the following elements:

- Sit upright on a stool that allows your knees to bend at 90 degrees when you are seated.
- Place your feet parallel to each other at shoulder width apart.
- Keep your torso upright at an angle of 90 degrees with your thighs.
- Rest your palms gently on your thighs with your arms bent naturally at the elbows.
- Tuck your chin in and allow your shoulders to relax.
- Draw your chest inward slightly and keep your back straight.
- Close your mouth and tip your tongue to the roof of your palate.

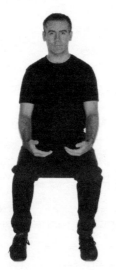
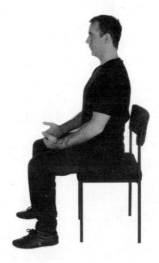

For most of the exercises you will perform them in a standing posture, if possible. It is therefore important that you get the standing posture correct as it is fundamental to all the exercises. Most of us have been conditioned to believe that correct posture involves sticking your chest out and arching your lower back. This in fact is not good posture as it curves the spine. Correct chi kung posture straightens and stretches the back and therefore allows the energy to flow smoothly along the spine.

You can experience the feeling of straightening your spine by lying on the floor with your feet flat on the ground and knees bent. When you press the arch of your back against the floor such that there is no space between the ground and your lower back, this means that you have straightened your spine. When standing in correct chi kung posture, your spine should feel somewhat similar.

When perfecting chi kung posture, at first it will not feel comfortable. All change involves initial discomfort and the more you practise, the more chi kung posture will bring comfort to you and your back. The main point of postural training is to relax in the various postures.

The following are the key principles of correct standing posture:

- Stand with your feet parallel to your shoulders, with your weight evenly distributed between each foot.
- Bend your knees and face forward in the same direction as your feet.
- Relax your hips. If you imagine that there is a tail coming from your tailbone, then tilt your sacrum as if you would be tucking that tail underneath your body. This feels unusual at first, but it effectively stretches the curve at the lower part of the spine.
- Relax your waist and avoid tensing the abdominal muscles.
- Stretch your back and suspend your head by imagining a weight hanging from the coccyx and a rope pulling up the crown of the head.
- Relax your shoulders and let them hang naturally, where they should drop and roll forward.

- Relax your armpits, elbows and wrists, allowing them to bend and hollow slightly.
- Relax your eyelids, leaving the eyes slightly open.
- Close your mouth and tip your tongue to the roof of your palate. This forms a connection between two important meridians in your body – the governing and conception vessels.
- Turn your hearing inwards so that you are free from outside interference.

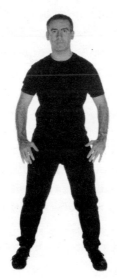

Correct Chi Kung Breathing

We are born with a natural ability to breathe properly. If you watch young children breathing, you will see their tummies expand more than their chests. However, as we get older we enter the illusion that proper breathing involves puffing out our chest and lifting our shoulders. This usually means that we are only breathing into our upper chest, which results in insufficient intake of oxygen for the brain and cells throughout our body.

The diaphragm is a sheet-like band of muscle that separates the chest from your abdomen. When the diaphragm relaxes, it moves up into the chest cavity, the lungs contract and air is forced out. When the diaphragm expands, it moves down into the abdominal cavity, pressing on the lower organs. If you are using the full capacity of your lungs, which is only possible with proper abdominal breathing, your blood receives sufficient oxygen, digestion is improved, your internal organs are strengthened, and lymph moves more efficiently through your lymphatic system. Proper breathing, therefore, has a profound impact on your immune system and contributes greatly to a sense of physical and emotional well-being.

There are many breathing methods used in chi kung training, but for the purposes of the Healing Code Chi Kung Programme, we will utilise natural abdominal respiration. Here you simply allow your abdomen to expand upon inhalation and contract upon exhalation. This breathing approach naturally increases your body's peristaltic (digestive) action and massages your internal organs. The key point about breathing is that it should be smooth and relaxed and generally 'circular'. Breathing should never be exaggerated or forced. This means that there should be a smooth and relaxed transition between inhalation and exhalation.

Take some time to practise this now. Placing your right hand on your abdomen, breathe in for three seconds, allowing your stomach to relax and expand. Breathing out for three seconds, gently allow your abdomen to fall. Take ten minutes to practise this technique.

If you have been habitually breathing incorrectly for a number of years, you must practise abdominal breathing frequently in order to retrain your body to accept this normal breathing pattern.

The Importance of Chi Kung Intention

Mental intention is the key element of chi kung that sets it apart from exercise systems of the Western world. It simply involves using visualisations to complement the exercises. Everybody has the ability to use mental intention. To prove this, consider the following:

1. What colour is your front door? On which side do you put the key?

2. Describe your favourite photograph.

In order to respond to the above you have to be able to create images in your mind. These images are visualisations and you will use this same ability to coordinate your mental intention when performing chi kung exercises.

The Three Steps to Learning Chi Kung Exercises

As you read the descriptions of the following exercises, you will notice that there are three stages that you need to perfect in order to practise chi kung correctly. These are 1) physical movement, 2) breathing and 3) mental intention.

You should concentrate on perfecting each stage in sequence. If initially you are not timing your breathing correctly or not focusing on the visualisations with deep intention, this is understandable. Just allow yourself the space and time to develop your awareness of the full exercise and it will come to you.

The Five Stages of Chi Kung Healing

When practising chi kung exercises, there are five primary stages of healing that occur through self-regulation therapy. The Healing Code Chi Kung Programme leads you through these five stages.

1. You increase your awareness of your body – physically, mentally and emotionally – and its current condition – One Through Ten Meditation.

2. You cleanse and purify your body's energetic fields to rid it of chi or energy stagnations and toxic pathogenic factors – purification exercises.

3. You strengthen and recharge your body to replenish the chi – organ-strengthening exercises.

4. You circulate the chi internally and externally throughout your body's entire energetic structure, moving any stagnant chi and strengthening the body – regulation exercise.

5. You dissipate any excess chi from your body by way of self-massage – dry skin brushing.

I have then included some exercises that I consider to be essential to health recovery, including chi kung walking, as well as an exercise to help you sleep.

As you begin learning the exercises you may also find it useful to have more visual guidance. If so, a Healing Code Chi Kung Programme instructional DVD is available at www.healing-code. com.

The Healing Code
Chi Kung Programme

Stage One

The One Through Ten (Tree) Meditation

We will begin the Healing Code Chi Kung Programme with arguably the most powerful chi kung meditation, commonly known as the Tree Meditation in China. The meditation is designed to relax both your mind and body. It builds and strengthens your energy and sets the tone for the Healing Code Chi Kung Programme by creating the desired mental and physical state for healing within your body.

Before you begin this exercise, set the ambiance of the environment you are going to work in. Either go to a very quiet place or put on some soft relaxation music. If you do use music, make sure you use the same music every time you perform the programme. This is because the music you play will soon become anchored to the mental and physical sense of well-being that you will achieve when practising. Before long you will be able to 'get into the zone' of mind and body relaxation simply by listening to this music.

It is important to familiarise yourself with the sequence of this meditation and initially you may do so by recording the script and playing it back when you are practising. So begin the exercise by standing or sitting in correct chi kung posture and then follow the counting format below.

Method

1. One is sun. Imagine placing a small golden sun on the front of your forehead. Feel the warmth of the sun's joyous glow melting

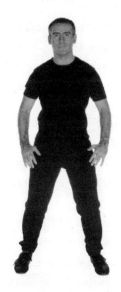 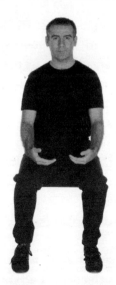

down the front of your body like warm oil, melting all tension and stress away down into the ground. Place a second golden sun on the back of your head. Feel a flowing sense of relaxation drifting down the back of your neck, taking all tension from your shoulders and dissolving all tension from the back of your body. Place a third sun on the top of your head, melting into your brain, relaxing your thoughts. You feel it melting down the centre of your body, dissolving all emotional and physical tension that was residing in your chest and abdomen. This sense of relaxation continues to flow down the centre of your legs and into the ground.

2. Two is shoe. Imagine your feet melting into the ground. Merging with the earth, your feet fuse in five directions: to the front, back, left, right and straight down. Visualise your body connecting with the earth.

3. Three is tree. Now visualise extending tree roots twice your body's height deep into the ground. The roots expand in the same five directions: to the front, back, both sides and down. This secures and roots your energy into the earth.

4. Four is core. Now imagine these roots extending even more deeply into the core of the planet. Visualise blue earth energy flowing into the roots. The energy enters and feeds your body just

as it would a tree. The energy flows up your legs, spine and over your head, then down your chest and enters into your abdomen in an area known as the 'Lower Dantian', which is your centre of physical energy. Visualise your abdomen filling up with powerful healing earth energy.

5. Five is alive. Now visualise this blue earth energy building up with such power that it starts to overflow into the centre of your chest like a mighty river of energy, dividing into two rivers, which flow down your arms and out through each palm into the earth.

6. Six is thick. Imagine the place where you are standing or sitting is being filled with energy so thick that it seems as if you are submerged in it. This is environmental energy and it fuses with the earth energy and your own energy to form one dynamic field of energy.

7. Seven is heaven. Now visualise divine or natural white healing energy flooding into your body from the top of your head. Imagine it filling your head area until it shines and floods down to your chest, where it again fills up your chest until it overflows down into your abdomen. You now visualise heavenly and earthly energies fusing within your body.

8. Eight is gate. Visualise each pore in your body opening up and drawing in the environmental energy with each inhalation of breath. Upon each exhalation imagine the centre core of your body vibrating and glowing like a bright light. This energises the centre core of your body and harmonises your energy with your breath.

9. Nine is shine. Now visualise your centre core becoming completely full of energy and shining so brightly out through your pores that it fills up the entire space around you with powerful white healing energy.

10. Ten is begin. Now realise that you are in physical, mental, emotional, energetic and spiritual harmony and you are ready to begin practice.

Stage Two – Purification Exercises

Purification exercises address what Chinese medicine calls chi stagnation. This is where energy is not moving properly and consequently illness or disharmony occurs. A wide variety of conditions have their roots in chi stagnation, including angina, coronary heart disease, depression and cancer. Chi stagnation can be caused by many different factors, but one of the primary ones is the repression of emotions. These exercises are also therefore for improving emotional well-being.

Pulling Down the Heavens Exercise

Method

1. Begin in correct chi kung posture. Hold the stance for approximately three minutes.

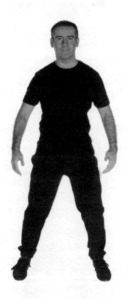

2. Inhale through your nose as you draw your arms to your sides, palms facing downwards. Visualise absorbing the energy from the earth and the environment around you.

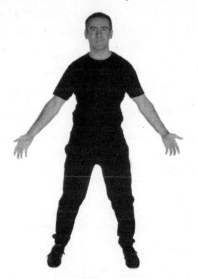

3. Continue inhaling as you turn your palms up to the sky and visualise grasping divine healing energy down from the heavens. Complete the breath inhalation with your palms facing the top of your head.

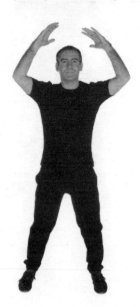

4. In a continuous smooth movement, draw your hands down the front of your body and visualise guiding the healing energy down-wards as you slowly exhale.

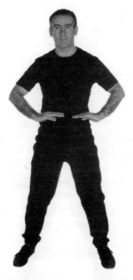

5. Repeat this sequence three times, visualising guiding the energy down the front, back and centre of your body.

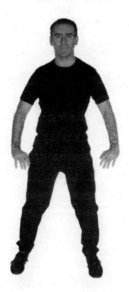

Counterswing – Chi Scattering Exercise

Method

1. Begin in correct chi kung posture.

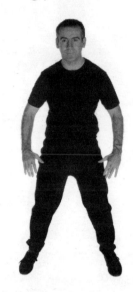

2. Inhale as you draw your arms up to the sides to form a T.

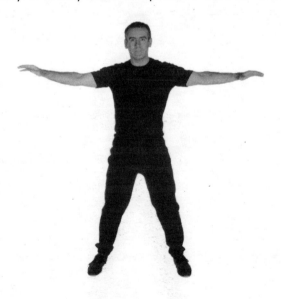

3. Breathe out as you turn to the left at the waist (not at the knees), swing your right arm up to the left and the left behind your back to the right. Your palms should be facing up when swinging out. At the end of the swing, extend and stretch out the fingers as if tossing a ball.

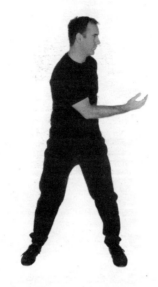

4. Breathe in as you allow your arms to drop and return to the T position.

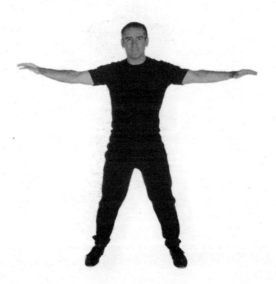

5. Breathe out as you turn to the right at the waist, swing your left arm up to the right and the right behind your back to the left. Your palm should be facing up when swinging out. At the end of the swing, extend and stretch out the fingers.

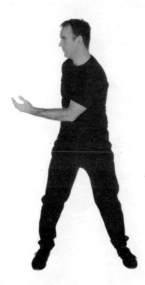

6. Turning at the waist to face the front, swing your left arm down and up to the left and the right back to the right to the level of your waist.

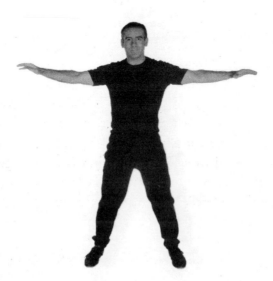

7. As you breathe in, imagine fresh clean energy being pumped up from the earth, through your feet, ankles, legs, hips and chest. As you breathe out, imagine grey, dirty, used energy being tossed out from your hands. With each breath out, the energy pushed out through the fingers becomes whiter and cleaner. Repeat this exercise for three to four minutes.

8. Finish by doing the Pulling Down the Heavens Exercise.

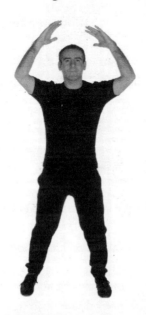

Stage Three – Organ-strengthening Exercises

Organ-strengthening exercises address what is seen as energetic and functional weaknesses in the internal organs, as well as the paths of energy that flow from the channels of each organ. Most of the exercises are named after the organ that is being helped. Organ deficiencies can occur for a variety of reasons such as overwork, overstress, prolonged over-indulgence and failure to get enough sleep. Organ-deficiency syndromes include such conditions as allergies, anaemia, anxiety, asthma, chronic fatigue and diabetes. These exercises will therefore prove very helpful for people with these conditions but will also be fundamental to the overall strengthening of your body so as to regain full health.

The Five Yang Organ Exercise

This exercise massages the internal digestive organs and strengthens the peristaltic action of the body's digestive system. Peristaltic action is the wave-like movement that occurs throughout your gastrointestinal tract – oesophagus, stomach, small intestine and colon – that helps move your food into your stomach, through your intestines and colon, and out through your rectum. This exercise also increases the capillary circulation by stimulating the autonomic nervous system.

The Five Yang Organ Exercise is therefore very beneficial for anyone encountering digestive problems such as constipation, chronic diarrhoea or irritable bowel syndrome.

Method

1. Stand in a wide stance, with your arms suspended by the sides of your body.
2. As you inhale, swing your arms up straight in front of your body and allow your hands to come into the chest. Expand the abdomen, with your mental intention on filling your lower abdomen with healing energy.
3. As you exhale, swing your arms back behind your body while compressing the abdomen down and inwards, imagining the circular flow of this energy in your lower abdominal area.

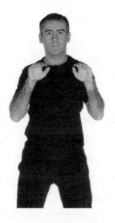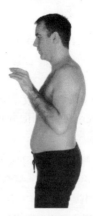

4. Continue to swing your arms back and forth at a comfortable pace with natural breathing. Allow the abdomen to expand and contract without forcing your breath.
5. Continue this repetition for at least 50 breaths, but work up to 250 breaths if you have problems with your digestion.

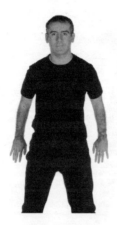 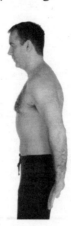

The Five Yin Organ Exercise

Each of the following exercises are designed to stimulate what are called the 'Yin' organs: Lungs, Kidneys, Liver, Heart and Spleen. In Chinese medicine, the Yin organs are responsible for producing, circulating and storing the fundamental energy in the body, the chi.

The Lung Exercise

The lungs are very important for the overall health of the body because they mix the chi with the blood and regulate the chi of the entire body. The chi of the outside world meets the chi of the human body in the lungs, and from there it is spread throughout the body. The health of the lungs manifests itself in the body hair and sweat glands, as well as the overall bodily health.

This exercise is designed to massage the lungs' tissues and nerves, as well as strengthen the entire lung organ and meridians. You practise this exercise to strengthen your respiratory system as well as to enhance your body's immune system.

Method

1. From normal posture,

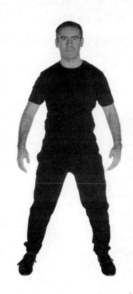

begin this exercise by moving your arms to the sides

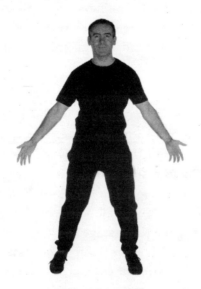

and stretching them up above your head.

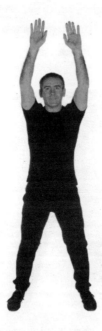

2. Allow your arms to float down in front of your chest at shoulder level, with the palms facing the floor.

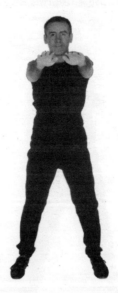

3. Inhale and bring the arms straight out to the sides. As you inhale, imagine absorbing bright white energy up from the ground through your palms. As the arms reach the sides of your body,

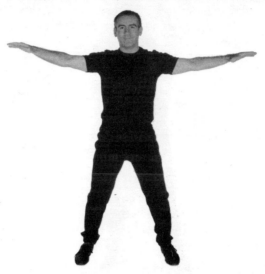

rotate your palms until they face upwards, whilst keeping your shoulders relaxed.

4. Now, while exhaling, bring the arms straight out in front of the body, palms still facing upwards.

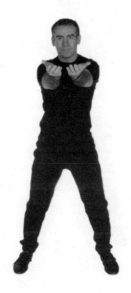

Visualise the energy flowing up along your arms and into your lungs, before settling into the abdomen.

5. Rotate your hands again, so that your palms are once again facing down and inhale as you again open your arms to repeat the sequence.

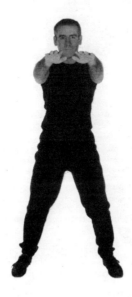

6. Repeat 20 times.

The Kidney Exercise

The kidneys are responsible for regulating the flow of water and fluids within the body, as well as for strong teeth and bones. Malfunctioning of the kidneys is particularly manifested through the ears. Thus hearing problems can be a symptom of kidney problems.

This exercise is designed to massage the kidneys' tissues and strengthen the entire organ, as well as the associated meridians. The twisting back and forth in this exercise stimulates the kidney organ, as the kidneys receive their blood supply from the abdominal aorta. This exercise is also used to strengthen the reproductive system, which is associated with kidney function in Chinese medicine.

Method

1. Upon completing the Lung Exercise, both hands are extended straight out in front of your body.

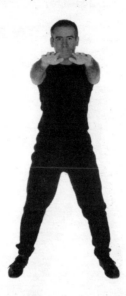

2. Inhale and drop your elbows, bringing your hands down in front of your lower abdomen.

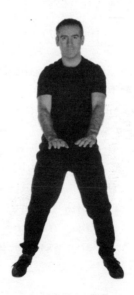

3. Exhale and shift the weight to the left. As the left palm wraps around your back, resting on the right kidney, the right hand extends towards the left.

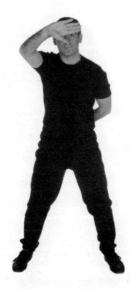

4. The right palm, facing outwards, begins to circle up in front of the face at eye level. Focus your eyes on the back of your hand as it moves across in front of your face.
5. Now shift your weight to the right side and begin leaning towards that side. Your eyes continue to follow the right palm as it circles downwards in front of your body.

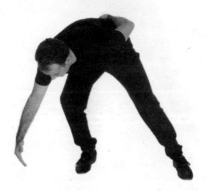

6. Exhale while shifting down. Bend your knees as you lean over and imagine scooping water with your right hand, palms now facing upwards. Keep your back relaxed and straight.

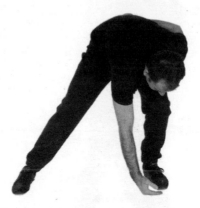

7. Allow your right arm to follow the movement of your body as you scoop across, slowly rising upright as you move to the left. As your palm begins to rise above your head, imagine the energy draining down your right arm like water, moving across your shoulders and down the left arm into the kidney.

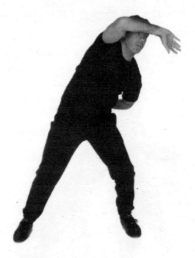

Repeat this side for ten repetitions.

8. Shift your weight on to the right leg.

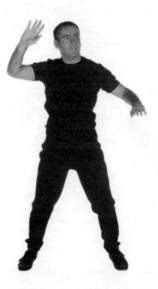

Now wrap your right hand around your back whilst you position your left hand in front of your face.

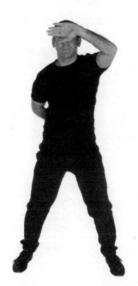

9. Begin to inhale and repeat for ten repetitions on this opposite side.

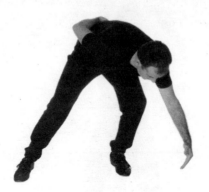

The Liver Exercise

This exercise is designed to massage the liver's tissues, as well as strengthen the entire organ and meridians. The liver in Chinese medicine is responsible for the smooth movement of the blood, bodily substances and, in general, of the chi throughout the body. Liver diseases are readily apparent through the eyes and the vision, and therefore many eye and vision difficulties are treated by treating the liver.

Malfunctioning of the liver can also manifest itself in emotional turmoil or digestion difficulties. The exercise mimics the similar action of throwing a punch and thereby simulates the expression and release of anger, which helps to regulate the emotional state.

Method

1. Upon completing the Kidney Exercise, place the right arm straight out in front of the body at shoulder level, palm facing down. Place the left hand by the left hip, palm facing upwards.

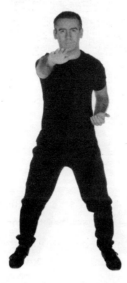

2. Simultaneously draw the right palm back and extend the left palm forward whilst inhaling. The left hand moves forward, passing the right hand (without touching), which is moving backwards.

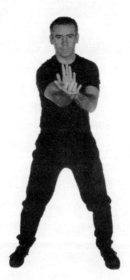

3. The hands continue in this motion using long and slow inhalation and exhalation.
4. Relax and repeat this sequence for 20 breaths. Feel the legs pumping and powering the push. Imagine the legs pumping green energy from the ground to the abdomen, up the back and out through the palms.

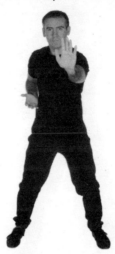

The Heart Exercise

This exercise is designed to massage the heart's tissues and nerves and strengthen the entire organ and meridians. This exercise is prescribed for many cardiac conditions, such as cardiac heart disease, hypertension, arrhythmia and rheumatic heart disease. You also practise this exercise to strengthen your circulatory system.

The heart is one of the most important organs within Chinese medicine. It circulates the blood and stores the human spirit. When the human spirit is properly nourished, it is in harmony with its surroundings and is happy. When the heart cannot sustain the spirit, the spirit becomes irrational and unfocused. It is worth noting that Chinese medicine knew about the heart's function to circulate blood thousands of years before English physiologist William Harvey 'discovered' the circulatory system in 1628.

The tongue and face are closely related to the heart, hence many diseases of the blood and heart can be diagnosed by examining the tongue and face.

Method

1. Upon completing the Liver Exercise, allow both hands to sink down in front of the lower abdomen.

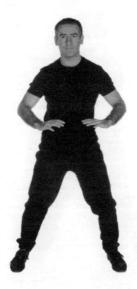

2. Imagine the hands embracing a fiery red ball, placing the right hand on top and the left hand on the bottom.

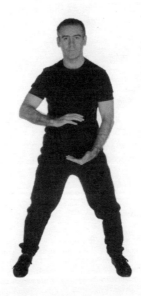

3. Exhale and twist to the left, simultaneously raising the left hand up over the head while extending the right hand towards the left.

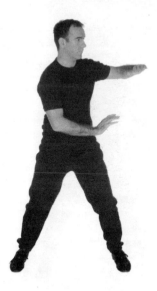

4. Continue pressing until both hands extend to the furthest point.

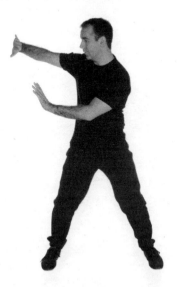

5. Inhale and turn the right hand upwards, imagine catching the ball as your body turns back to the centre, where the right hand is positioned in front of the navel.

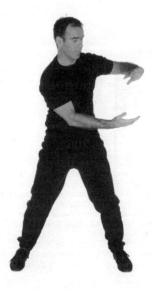

The left hand simultaneously turns so that the palm faces the centre of the right hand as you continue to imagine holding the fiery red ball.

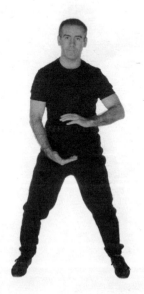

6. From this central position, you now exhale and twist to the right, simultaneously raising the right hand up over the head while extending the left hand towards the right.

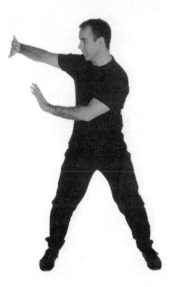

Imagine catching the ball again as you return your body to the centre.

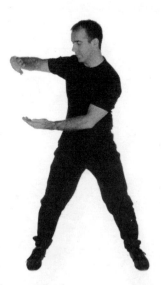

7. Repeat ten times on each side.

The Spleen Exercise

This exercise is designed to massage the spleen's tissues, as well as strengthen the entire organ and meridians. This exercise is therefore prescribed to enhance the function of the digestive system. The spleen is considered vital in Chinese medicine as it transforms food into blood and chi and regulates the digestion. In Chinese medicine the spleen is also seen to govern the muscles, flesh and limbs. Weak limbs may indicate problems with the spleen. The mouth and lips are also closely related to the spleen as is the sense of taste.

Method

1. Upon completing the Heart Exercise, assume a standing posture and allow your body to relax and breathe naturally.
2. Exhale and slowly turn to the left as you allow your relaxed arms to swing with the movement.
3. Inhale as you return to the centre, and with a continuous smooth movement, continue to swing to the right, exhaling and using your waist as an axle. Allow your head to follow the direction of the swinging arms and visualise golden yellow energy spiralling up your legs from the ground.
4. Repeat ten times on each side.

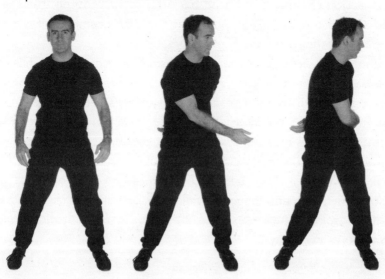

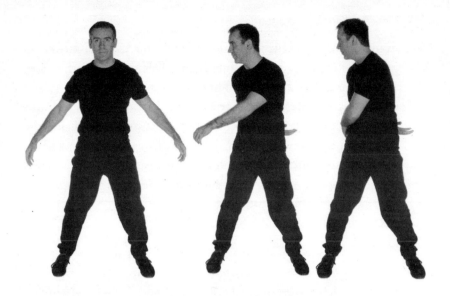

Stage Four – Regulation Exercise

Kwan Gong Stroking Beard (Microcosmic Orbit) Meditation

This is the classic Taoist meditation method for refining, raising and circulating internal energy via the 'orbit', formed by the 'governing channel' from perineum up along the spine to the head and the 'conception channel' from head back down the centre of the chest and abdomen to perineum. Activating the microcosmic orbit is a key step that leads to more advanced practices.

Chinese medics believe that microcosmic orbit meditation fills the reservoirs of the governing and conception channels with energy, which is then distributed to all the major organ-energy meridians, thereby energising the internal organs. It draws abundant energy up from the sacrum into the brain, thereby enhancing cerebral circulation of blood and stimulating secretions of vital neurochemicals. This is probably one of the best of all Chinese medical methods for cultivating health and longevity while also 'opening the three passes' to higher spiritual awareness. You should practise this meditation for 15 minutes each day.

Method

1. The first step is to still your mind, calm your body and regulate your breath. With this settled mind, sit or stand alone in a quiet room, senses shut and eyelids lowered.
2. Turn your attention within and visualise a ball of energy in the umbilical region. Within it is a point of golden light, clear and bright, immaculately pure.
3. Holding your hands about a foot apart, level with your navel, focus attention on this area of your abdomen until you 'feel' this ball of energy glowing in this region.

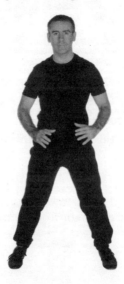

The breath through your nose will naturally become light and subtle, going out and in evenly and finely, continuously and quietly, gradually becoming slighter and subtler.

4. When the feeling is stable and the energy there is full, using your mind and guiding with your hands, draw the energy down to the perineum and visualise this energy rising up the spine to the back of your skull – known as the 'jade pillow'. Your hands rise up the front of your chest as your mental intention draws this energy along the spine.
5. When this energy passes through the jade pillow, press the tongue against the palate. Feel the energy pass over the skull and begin to travel down the centre of your forehead.

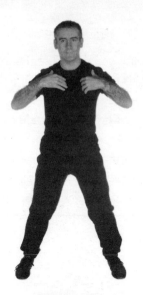

6. Next, focus attention on drawing the energy down to the area between the eyebrows and draw the energy forwards from the mid-brain and out through the point between the brows. This can occasionally cause a tingling or throbbing sensation. This is a positive sensation as energy blockages are clearing.

7. Now, guiding your hands down as if stroking a beard (hence the name of the exercise), visualise the energy sinking down through the palate and tongue and down the front centre of your chest. This may

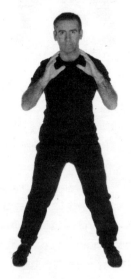

feel as though there is cool water going down your windpipe. Do not swallow; let it go down by itself, bathing the bronchial tubes.

8. From the centre of the chest – the heart, draw it down through the mid-region into the solar plexus, past the navel and down to the umbilical region where we began.

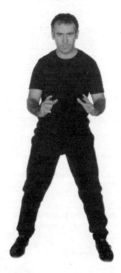

Then begin another cycle and repeat.

9. Breathe naturally with your abdomen, and don't worry whether energy moves up or down on inhalation or exhalation; coordinate the flow of breath and energy in whatever manner suits you best.

If you practise this way for a long time, you will soon complete a whole cycle of the visualisation without any mental effort. You can practise this inner work continuously throughout the day, whether walking, standing still, sitting or lying down. The vital energy will circulate harmoniously within, and consequently Chinese medics believe many chronic physical ailments will begin to rectify themselves.

Stage Five

Dry Skin Brushing

Perform dry skin brushing once a day just before showering. The benefits of dry skin brushing include:

1. It will help to remove dead layers of skin, improving the health of your skin.
2. It will increase the blood circulation to the skin and the underlying organs and tissues.
3. It will improve lymphatic drainage of your entire body.
4. It will help your skin's ability to eliminate toxic materials.
5. It will improve oxygenation and reflexive stimulation of your entire body.

Your skin is your body's largest organ. It receives one-third of all the blood that is circulated in your body and should eliminate about one-third of all your body's waste each day. Your skin acts as the main organ of detoxification, when other organs involved with the elimination of toxins are overburdened, the skin will become overloaded and this will show as eruptions or discharges.

If, therefore, your blood is full of toxic materials, the condition of the skin will almost always reflect this, with problems such as eczema or boils. Skin problems can indicate problems with the organs that eliminate toxins from the body, such as the liver or colon. So skin problems reflect internal ill health. Chronic skin problems are an outward reflection of a problem that is inside the body.

For this exercise you can use a soft, dry bath brush, but it is best to purchase a proper dry-skin brush from your local health shop. Dry skin brushing is usually done just before a bath or shower and you never allow the brush to get wet.

Method

1. Standing unclothed, lightly stroke the brush across the top of the foot to the knee. Always brush towards the heart.
2. Continue lightly stroking the entire body in long, light, smooth strokes, up the arms and legs. You only need to brush each surface once: one stroke for the front of the lower leg, one for the inside, one for the outside and one for the back of the leg. It only takes about four strokes from the foot to the knee.

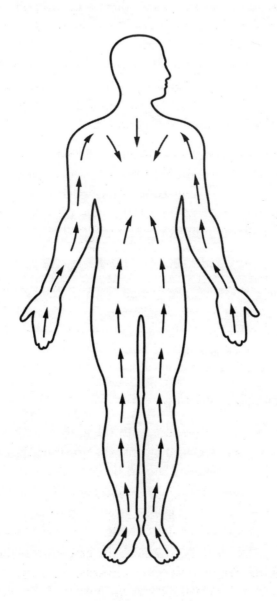

The correct technique for dry skin brushing

3. Brush the upper legs and arms in the same manner. It takes only six strokes for the upper leg and four strokes from the hand to the shoulder.
4. The trunk is lightly stroked with the target being the liver, which is under the ribs on the right side. You do not brush your face, tender or sensitive areas, or irritated areas where there are cuts or scrapes.

Essential Cancer Healing Exercises

The following exercises have been used extensively to support cancer recovery. They can, however, be used to treat a variety of other conditions and chi kung walking therapy in particular should become a part of your daily exercise routine no matter what condition you are recovering from.

Dispelling the Filth and Rebuilding the Energy Meditation

The Dispelling the Filth and Rebuilding the Energy Meditation is generally prescribed for those recovering from stomach, pancreatic, ovarian, uterine, cervical, bladder, prostate, colon or rectal cancer. Patients with these conditions should practise these prescriptions four to six times a day.

Method – Dispelling the Filth

1. Begin from a sitting posture, with the eyes closed and the body relaxed, the tongue placed against the upper hard palate behind the teeth. Your breathing should be natural and even.
2. Perform the One Through Ten Meditation (see page 222).
3. Inhale and imagine healing light entering in through the nose and the top of your head. Imagine and feel this healing light penetrating and filling all of the specific cancer area, illuminating and vibrating the tissues and cells.
4. Exhale and imagine energy beginning to whirl clockwise throughout the entire body. Starting above the area where the illness is focused, imagine energy whirling in through the tissues of the cancer, circulating clockwise on a horizontal plane, moving downward through the entire body, building momentum as it flows downward.

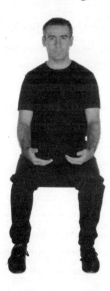

5. Imagine the whirling energy flowing throughout the internal tissues. As it moves through the internal organs and channels, the whirling energy begins absorbing the noxious heat and filthy energy from the diseased tissues, transforming it into wind and dispelling it out of your body and into the earth.
6. Practise for ten repetitions.
7. Perform the Pulling Down the Heavens Exercise for three breaths in order to further cleanse and purify the tissues.

Method – Rebuilding the Energy

1. Next, imagine and feel the white healing light vibrating and flowing upward from the centre of the planet into your body, penetrating and completely saturating the body's tissues and cells with divine healing light.
2. Gently imagine drawing the energy into the specific cancer area. As the divine healing energy enters the cancer area, it becomes transformed into a form of healing wind. This wind rebuilds and strengthens the body's tissues and cells as it internally circulates within the body in a horizontal anticlockwise direction. This wind spirals up the body through the internal organs and channels, and is expelled out through the mouth.

3. Practise for ten repetitions.
4. To end this meditation, focus the attention on your lower abdomen and perform the Pulling Down the Heavens Exercise for three breaths. Imagine that vital energy is returning back to its origin in the lower abdomen – the 'lower dan tien'. Place both hands on the lower abdomen and imagine the chi collecting and settling in the area.
5. End the prescription by resting undisturbed for 15 minutes.

Chi Kung Walking Therapy

You may be surprised that a simple exercise such as walking can do so much to heal your body, but modern Western science is only just beginning to understand how powerful an exercise walking is.

There are many different styles of chi kung walking exercises. The system we are going to use is less elaborate than some systems but equally as effective. Try to perform chi kung walking exercises outdoors in the countryside or in a parkland area where the air is cleaner. Always dress to keep yourself warm when walking. You should aim to walk for 30 minutes to an hour each day.

Method – Physical Movement

1. When you begin walking, step forward and touch down with your heel first and with your toes pointing up.

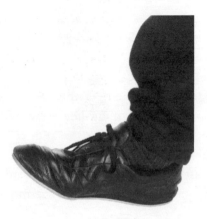

2. Roll your foot down until your toes touch the ground, keeping your knees slightly bent.

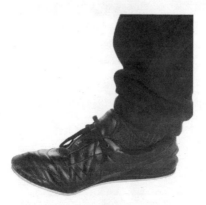

3. As you step, sway your arms from side to side, coordinating with your steps. When you step forward with your right foot, sway your arms to the right.

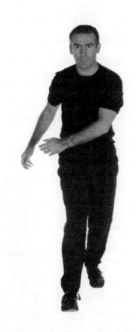

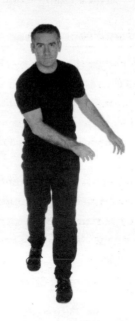

Sway your arms to the left as you step forward with the left foot. Keep your arms and hands relaxed.

The rhythm and speed of your chi kung walking is important. For conditions above the diaphragm but below the neck – such as lung disease – your speed should be 90 steps per minute. For conditions of the digestive system, liver and gall bladder, your speed should be 60 steps per minute. Finally, for conditions of the lower abdominal area – kidneys and bladder – as well as brain conditions, your pace should be 40 steps per minute.

Breathing

Inhale as you step forward with your left foot and exhale as you step forward with your right foot.

Mental Intention

As you are walking, imagine that the diseased area of the body you are working on is vibrating with each step. Visualise the diseased cells and tissues breaking up and flowing down your body and legs then scattering from your feet into the ground.

The Old Man and the Tide Pool Exercise

This exercise was introduced to the West by Dr Her Yue Wong in the 1970s. Dr Wong believed that this exercise was the most effective way of releasing negative emotional energy from the body. It therefore fits alongside the emotional element of the Healing Code and is used to 'purge' your body of stagnant emotions, in particular sorrow, anger and worry.

As well as physical movement, mental intention and breathing, this exercise incorporates powerful healing sounds, which function to express and release these toxic emotions. As you will be making noise during this exercise, you might wish to perform it in a quiet, secluded area. If you feel self-conscious when first performing this exercise, bear in mind that it is the most powerful emotional healing exercise in the Healing Code.

Chi kung frequently uses sound as part of treatment. When your body experiences any type of sound, the cell tissues respond to the tone frequency. According to Jerry Alan Johnson, when sound waves vibrate in the body, crystalline structures within the tissues transform the vibration into pulsed currents. These currents are then conducted to the various corresponding organs and glands, depending on the frequency and amplitude of the incoming wave signal. Sound, or tone resonances, have been used for centuries as a healing tool in chi kung. Of course, in more recent times conventional medicine has adopted sound therapy. High-intensity ultrasound is used routinely to treat soft-tissue injuries, such as strains, tears and associated scarring. The heating and agitation are believed to promote rapid healing through increased circulation. Strongly focused, high-intensity, high-frequency ultrasound can also be used to physically destroy certain types of tumour, as well as gallstones and other types of calculi. Developing new treatment applications for ultrasound is an active area of medical research.

Method

1. Begin the exercise from a standing posture, with both feet facing forward, shoulder width apart. Inhale and imagine healing energy

filling up your lungs. As you inhale, separate both arms to the side of the body, forming a T shape.

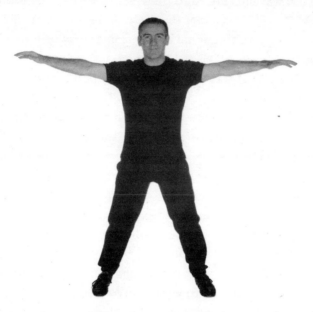

2. Bend over and exhale whilst making the sound 'Shhhhhhhh' – much like you would hush a baby. As you exhale, imagine toxic energy flowing down each arm and into the ground. Both arms should swing from one side to the other, crisscrossing, whilst making the purging sound.

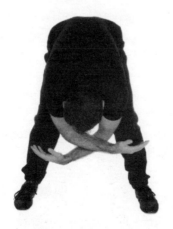

3. Inhale as you slowly return to an upright position, allowing your spine to roll back up vertebra by vertebra as you raise your arms to the sides

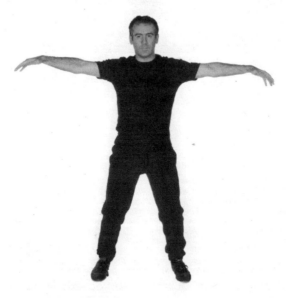

and above your head.

4. Imagine grasping healing energy with soft fists, as if gently holding two tiny birds.

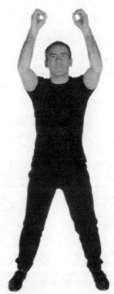

5. As you exhale, descend your hands to shoulder level.

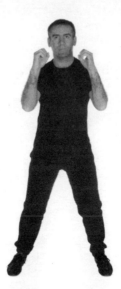

Focus your mind on the centre of your chest and imagine toxic energy releasing from your heart as you exhale half your breath whilst making a 'Haa-a-a-a-a' sound.

6. Now as you release the remaining breath, allow your hands to drop from shoulder level to your hips and make a 'Who-o-o-o-o' sound.

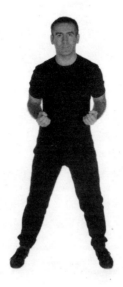

7. Move your arms up again to the sides

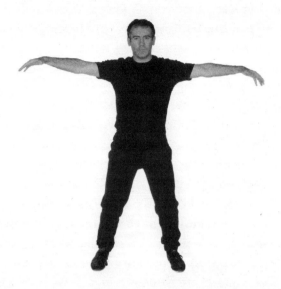

and above your head and repeat steps four to six three times.

8. This completes one set of the exercise. You should perform 36 sets in total, which should take approximately 25 minutes. Perform this exercise once a day for a total of five consecutive days.

Chi Kung and Sleep

There is a lot of confusion about the importance of sleep. Some self-help books on the market promote the idea of sleeping no more than five hours a night, and some well-known historical world figures survived with very little sleep. However, just because they were world leaders doesn't mean that they were healthy, and most of them were not. It was Napoleon Bonaparte who famously said about the hours of sleep required, 'Six for the man, seven for the woman and eight for the fool.' However, Napoleon suffered from a long string of ailments, including depression, epilepsy, scabies, neurodermatitis, migraine, painful urination, chronic hepatitis and stomach cancer. Napoleon was also just 51 when he died.

With busy lives, sleep is often the first thing that is sacrificed.

However, if you are recovering from illness, you need to be aware that it is during sleep that your body restores itself.

With the help of this book, you have programmed your mind for health, emotionally cleansed, cleaned out toxins and fuelled your body with superfoods. But it is actually during your sleeping hours that your body takes advantage of all these massively helpful steps. The sleeping hours are when you take these building blocks of health and restore your body. While you are sleeping your body is resting and refuelling. Your blood pressure drops, and your heartbeat and metabolism slow. This enables the cells in your body to repair themselves and for your body to create new cells including in your immune system. Poor sleep weakens immune function and reduces the number of killer cells that combat germs and cells that divide too rapidly, as well as cancer cells. Further studies have shown that chronic sleep deprivation also contributes to gastro-intestinal problems, heart disease and a host of other medical conditions.

You know you are getting good sleep when you wake refreshed in the morning. If you are not waking refreshed, then you are probably not getting enough sleep, or else your sleep quality is poor. If you are waking frequently during the night to go to the bathroom, or are having such vivid dreams that they are disturbing your sleep, then this obviously affects your sleep quality. This will impinge on the strengthening of your immune system, which should be taking place at night-time.

Chi kung practices fully recognise the importance of sleep and use exercise to enhance sleep. In general the exercises in the Healing Code Chi Kung Programme put you in harmony with nature. This means that when practised at night-time, they will help to bring you into a state of quiescence and calm. When performed in the morning, they will invigorate you physically for the day ahead.

You should aim to be in bed with the lights out at 10 p.m. If you are not used to getting to bed this early, move your bedtime back by half an hour every week until you are going to sleep at 10 p.m. This means that activities that you are used to doing in the evening, such as watching TV, should also be discontinued half an hour earlier each week. Very soon your bedtime will be 10 p.m. and you will be more in harmony with the earth's natural sleeping time for a human. Consequently, falling asleep will become easier and rest will be deeper and more rewarding.

You should also be sure that your bedroom is conducive to sleep. Remove all the clutter and make sure that your bed is soft and comfortable. Make sure that you have soft sheets and surround yourself with pillows. It is also a good idea not to overstimulate your brain before attempting to fall asleep. This means switching off the TV at least 20 minutes before retiring. If you are going to read in bed, make sure you give yourself time to wind down after reading.

With the Healing Code Nutrition Plan, you will already be avoiding caffeinated beverages. If you do need to drink before bed, consider a soothing mug of camomile tea, which is conducive to sleep. Avoid having too much to drink before bedtime, however, as this is likely to interrupt your sleep in order to go to the bathroom.

If you have problems with your sleeping, you can also practise this chi kung exercise, which is particularly effective at inducing a deep sleep. This should be performed sitting on your bed with pillows at your back which you can fall on to as you drift into sleep.

Chi Kung Sleep Exercise

Method

1. Clap your hands and rub them together to draw heat from your heart.

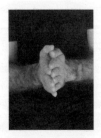

2. Massage your lower back in the kidney area, known as 'mingmen' or the 'gate of vitality', 36 times.

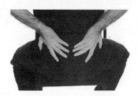

3. Place both hands over your mingmen area and, during three breaths, imagine sending chi from your hands into your kidneys.
4. Repeat two or three times.
5. Place your right ankle on your left knee and your right hand on your navel. Now with your left hand gently massage the sole of the right foot until you start to fall asleep.

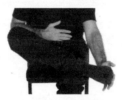

In Summary

- Follow a gradual approach to chi kung exercise and gather the benefits of exercise without taking yourself to exhaustion. Begin slowly, and as your strength and stamina increase, gradually increase the duration and the pace of your activity.
- Practise chi kung every day. To maximise the health benefits, it is important to be consistent. Make sure to include chi kung exercise as a vital part of your schedule.
- Maximise your comfort and safety. Be sure to keep warm and wear clothes and shoes that move comfortably with you. Always exercise in a safe location and at a comfortable pace.
- Challenge yourself. Set sensible goals and celebrate every success!
- Enjoy chi kung. Where possible, invite friends and family to join in.

So we have now looked at the five pillars of the Healing Code – mind, emotion, nutrition, detoxification and exercise. You may have already performed many of the exercises and tasks at this stage. Great! The key to the success of the Healing Code is to take what you have learned and to put it into action. As the ancient Chinese proverb says, 'A journey of a thousand miles begins with one step.' It's time to fully implement the Healing Code programme.

CHAPTER SEVEN

Living Your Dream

I don't think it's possible to face a life-challenging illness and not be changed by it. For many people, such an event is the call to action that had been needed in order to make significant changes in their lives. Maintaining a positive psychological framework, balanced emotional state, healthy eating habits, being toxin-free and enjoying regular exercise have got to be a powerful catalyst for hugely positive life changes. I trust you now realise that implementing the lessons of the Healing Code is in fact a gift that goes beyond addressing your health issues. It goes right to the core of who you are, encouraging the development of inner self-confidence, positive self-image and of course a significantly increased sense of well-being. It helps you to reclaim your life. The Healing Code therefore opens the door to realising your full and true potential.

For years I suffered on in a loathsome career in which I could not fulfil any sense of self-expression or life purpose. Making any real changes was always something that I would look at 'tomorrow'. Of course, unless a real sense of urgency is created, tomorrow never comes. The illness and, more to the point, my reaction to that temporary loss of health completely changed my life – for the better! In that sense it has been a great blessing.

The tools necessary to implement the Healing Code are possessed within all of us. By making the Healing Code an integral part of your life, you can use it to achieve many goals that you would have postponed in the past. In my clinics, I have witnessed clients who encounter health challenges soon develop a profound self-belief that had not been present before. These fantastic people develop a strong sense of life purpose, which grants benefits that are not only physical.

Through consistency, visualisation and positive determination, you too can succeed in not only achieving a total health recovery but also turning your life around completely. Remember, it's not the cards we are dealt that matters, but rather how we play them. Aiming for the absolute best, exceeding your expectations and reaching for the highest standards are all ultimately always your choice. We all have the power and indeed the gift to create our own sense of life's meaning.

Dreams can and do become reality. Goals can also become bigger, bolder and more exciting. The more concrete and vividly you visualise these goals, imagining what exactly they will feel like when you experience them, the sooner you can begin to actually live the dream. Grab life with both hands. Of course, it involves effort on your part. Realising your full potential always requires commitment, self-discipline, enthusiasm and inner strength. It also requires a sense of joy and fun. If something is worth achieving, it should be enjoyable in the process.

The key to the Healing Code's success is to take what you have learned from the book and put it all into action. There are a number of exercises to perform and principles to implement. If you haven't done so already, go back to Chapter Two and start working through each exercise and chapter in the order in which they are presented. Take responsibility for your successful full recovery. Create a sense of momentum and celebrate (in a healthy way) all improvements in your health. Cultivate an attitude of gratitude, and as you progress each day, recognise that each step forward brings you closer to your goals of total health recovery and beyond.

I have done my best to pass on the principles and tools you can use to achieve powerful health benefits. They have worked for me and countless others, and they can work for you as well. As you practise the techniques in this book and fully implement the Healing Code, I want to make just one small request. When you have achieved a complete and total health recovery, use your own success story to inspire and motivate others who may experience similar challenges to those you encountered and overcame.

Life is a gift, and all of us have the responsibility to give something back. Your words of encouragement can truly make a huge difference. Be part of the Healing Code community and submit your own health success story to dermot@healing-code.com.

Until I hear from you, I would like to send you a famous Irish blessing:

> May the roads rise to meet you,
> May the wind be always at your back,
> May the sun shine warm upon your face,
> The rain fall soft upon your fields,
> And until we meet again,
> May God support you in the palm of His hand.

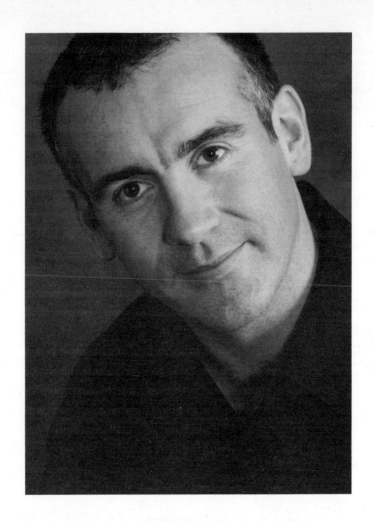

Spend the day with Dermot O'Connor

If you would like to join Dermot O'Connor at one of his Healing Code Workshops in the UK and Ireland or take part in Healing Code Practitioner Training visit *www.healing-code.com* or telephone +44 (0)871 218 0300 (UK) or +353 (0)1 667 2222 (Ireland).

Bibliography

Armstrong, Lance, *It's Not About the Bike: My Journey Back to Life* (Yellow Jersey Press, 2001)

Baillie-Hamilton, Paula, *Stop the 21st Century Killing You* (Vermilion, 2005)

Batmanghelidj, F., *Water for Health, for Healing, for Life: You're Not Sick, You're Thirsty!* (Warner Books, New York, 2003)

Callahan, Roger J., *Tapping the Healer Within: Using Thought-field Therapy to Instantly Conquer Your Fears, Anxieties and Emotional Distress* (Contemporary Books, 2000)

Campbell, T. Colin, and Campbell II, Thomas M., *The China Study* (Benbella Books, 2005)

Colbert, Don, *Deadly Emotions* (Nelson Books, 2003)

Coleman, Daniel, and the Dalai Lama, *Destructive Emotions* (Bantam Books, 2004)

Collins, Sean, and Draper, Rhoda, *The Key Model: a New Strategy for Cancer Recovery* (Ardagh Clinic, 2004)

Cousins, Norman, *Anatomy of an Illness* (W. W. Norton & Co., New York, 2005)

Fitzgerald, Patricia, *The Detox Solution: the Missing Link to Radiant Health, Abundant Energy, Ideal Weight and Peace of Mind* (Ebrandedbooks.com, 2001)

Frantzis, B. K., *Opening the Energy Gates of Your Body: Chi Gung for Lifelong Health* (Frog Ltd, 2006)

Hicks, Angela, and Hicks, John, *Healing Your Emotions: Discover Your Five Element Type and Change Your Life* (HarperCollins, 1999)

Hitchcox, Lee, *Long Life Now* (Nelson's Books, 1996)

Johnson, Jerry Alan, *Chinese Medical Qigong Therapy* (Redwing Book Company, 2000)

Koenig, Harold G., and Cohen, Harvey Jay, *The Link Between Religion and Health: Psychoneuroimmunology and the Faith Factor* (Oxford University Press Inc., 2002)

Larre, Claude, and de la Vallée, Elizabeth, *Chinese Medicine from the Classics: the Seven Emotions – Psychology and Health in Ancient China* (China Books, 1996)

Levy, Thomas E., *Optimal Nutrition for Optimal Health* (Keats Publishing, 2001)

Liang, Shou-Yu, and Wu, Wen-Ching, *Qigong Empowerment* (Way of the Dragon Ltd, 1996)

Martin, Paul, *The Sickening Mind: Brain, Behaviour, Immunity and Disease* (Flamingo, 1998)

Mazo, Ellen, *The Immune Advantage: How to Boost Your Immune System* (Rodale International, 2003)

McKenna, Paul, *Change Your Life in 7 Days* (Harmony, 2005)

Murphy, Joseph, *The Power of Your Subconscious Mind* (Bantam, New York, 2001)

Pert, Candace B., *Molecules of Emotion: Why You Feel the Way You Do* (Pocket Books, 1999)

Pitchford, Paul, *Healing with Whole Foods: Asian Traditions and Modern Nutrition* (North Atlantic Books, 2002)

Plant, Jane, and Tidey, Gill, *The Plant Programme: Eating for Better Health* (Virgin Books, 2005)

Quillin, Patrick, *Beating Cancer with Nutrition* (Nutrition Times Press Inc, 2005)

Rossi, Ernest Lawrence, *The Psychobiology of Mind-Body Healing: New Concepts of Therapeutic Hypnosis* (W. W. Norton & Co., New York, 1994)

Schwartz, Anna L., *Cancer Fitness* (Simon and Schuster, 2005)

Siegel, Bernie S., *Peace, Love and Healing: the Path the Self-Healing* (Rider and Co., 1999)

Swank, Roy Laver, and Brewer Dugan, Barbara, *The Multiple Sclerosis Diet Book: a Low-fat Diet for the Treatment of MS* (Bantam Books, 1987)

Vale, Jason, *The Juice Master's Slim 4 Life: Freedom from the Food Trap* (HarperCollins, 2002)

Wilcox, Bradley, Wilcox, Craig, and Suzuki, Makoto, *The Okinawa Way: How to Improve Your Health and Longevity Dramatically* (Mermaid Books, 2001)